As you encounter Jerrod Sessler's challenges and victories in "Five Percent Chance," you will grow to love and appreciate him as I do. I was privileged to first meet Jerrod in 2002 when he attended Health Minister Training at Hallelujah Acres. I enjoyed experiencing firsthand his enthusiasm and passion for helping others as we shared the stage at seminars and appeared on national television together. Jerrod is motivated by the love of God. He has a zeal for knowledge of both the Word of God and health as he seeks to empower others to take control of their health. He will lead you on the pathway to optimal health as he shares his journey with you.

Olin Idol, N.D., C.N.C., Vice-President of Health
Hallelujah Acres, Inc.
Author of Pregnancy, Children and The Hallelujah Diet

A few years ago Jerrod shared with me that he had survived a deadly cancer but was determined to fight it—naturally. Shortly before this conversation, a young lady in our office had died of cancer after going through horrendous treatments. The word "cancer" got my attention. So did the word "naturally." Jerrod shared that he basically gave up processed foods. He reminded me, "Jesus ate off the land." I had that extra ten pounds of weight I had been carrying around for years. I gave it a try and the pounds melted off. I slept better, I was more alert, and I was toxin free. Eating like Jesus and Jerrod has been a liberating lifestyle change for me.

Melanie Bergeron, Chairwoman
Two Men and a Truck/International

I want to take this opportunity to thank you from the bottom of my heart for the thoughtful guidance, encouragement, advice and support you gave me nearly five years ago when I first went on the Hallelujah Diet and Lifestyle. I was trying to recover from a list of life threatening illnesses, including: advanced congestive heart failure with atrial fibrillation; high blood pressure; severe seizures that almost took my life and played havoc with my mind; arthritis;, digestive problems; and a number of other health problems that made life almost not worth living. Every health problem just went away, as well as seventy pounds and eight inches off the waist, on the Hallelujah Diet. Knowing your family has been such a godsend to me. The weekly meetings that you and your lovely wife and children have had for me and many other people have probably been the difference between success and failure for many of us. I will never be able to thank you enough, my dear friend.

John Matthews
Thriving at 87. You can too!

Jerrod Sessler is a walking miracle. The fact that he is still on this earth is a testimony to the healing power of God and the smart lifestyle changes made by Jerrod. I've never known another individual who can make and set a goal, then focus his sights on that goal for success. I guess when you're faced with something like cancer, your priorities tend to get in focus pretty quick. I've learned about leadership, goal setting, mentoring, and healthy living from Jerrod. He was given only a five percent chance. Jerrod refused to sit back and believe what he was told and turned his five percent chance into one hundred percent success.
Loran Lichty, Pastor, Friend, Connector
LoranLichty.com

Jerrod's story of survival has been an inspiration to many. I admire his passion for educating people to help them make more informed choices to improve their health and the quality of their lives.
Jeff Rogers
Author, "Vice Cream" (www.vicecream.com)

Jerrod was an inspiration of faith when I was diagnosed with melanoma in 2006. His attitude towards life is a gift to any person who is battling with a difficult situation.
Alan Furmanski, Publisher and Writer of health books in Spanish

I am so grateful for the influence Jerrod and his family has had on my life. Among other things I am enjoying increased energy and health along with a wealth of information that continues to help vitalize my body & life.
Mark Yokers, Principal
Puget Sound Window Maintenance, Inc.

I met Jerrod in 2002 in Washington, D.C. We have been friends since that day. His story and faith have inspired me to face many obstacles. I enjoyed reading every word!
Michael Townsend -Business Consultant, Knoxville, Tennessee

The underlying message of the information Jerrod has collected in this book is one of hope. Due to Jerrod and Nikki's generosity of time, information, and know-how, I have been given the opportunity to succeed with this life-changing diet.
Heidi Slater
Raw Food Blog Author

Jerrod and I met several years ago at a seminar in North Carolina. He is a walking example of the results that are possible when we eat the diet we were created to eat. We can thrive with our health! Through his amazing healing journey, he has gained a great amount of knowledge that can help everyone. I highly recommend this book.
Paul Nison, Raw Food Author and Chef
PaulNison.com

Jerrod's "Cancer story" stands as a remarkable contrast of "life and Life." Because time is only relevant in the absence of eternity, the disease which is life threatening for many serves instead as a cause for celebration in God's servant Jerrod. Though the challenges of life continue, we are reminded how the promise of eternal Life has remained the same, and within our grasp, for two thousand years. Jerrod's sense of peace with his cancer experience is easy to explain...his "Life" is eternal, and was never threatened in the first place.
Steve Wadlington
President, WIN Home Inspection

Jerrod is definitely a unique leader who's example helps point us to a healthier lifestyle. Thanks to Jerrod, we realize how important it is to continue the education about diet and lifestyle choices and their impact on our health. Jerrod's story is nothing short of miraculous. He has been blessed with a faith and trust in God that is awesome to witness. His example, which is clearly demonstrated within "Five Percent Chance," has challenged us and our staff to widen our perspective on how our lifestyle choices really do have a direct impact on our health.
Dr. Jim & Lynn Coleman
Seahurst Dental Design

Five Percent Chance: Winning the Cancer Race will resonate with readers because it touches on two critical issues that our society, and this world, wrestles with today: the lack of health, well-being and spirituality, and the absence of a God-directed life. The author shares his secrets on how to obtain both optimal health and a heart at peace. The reader is sure to be touched as Jerrod tells his story about being diagnosed with cancer, which led him from sadness and fear to restoration and renewal.
Keefe J. McClung
Manager for a Fortune 500 Company

I came across Jerrod Sessler's story while researching case studies about raw food diets and their frequent association with physical healing. His testimony about recovering from cancer is one of the most inspiring ones I've ever read. The best part about Jerrod is his genuine concern for people and his willingness to let others peer into his private life while sharing important (and potentially life-saving) information. His personal, ongoing experience with nutritional excellence and its profound effects upon personal health is a must read for anyone who really wants to understand the simple, yet powerful way to genuine and lasting wellness.

Joe Farinaccio
Publisher, Living Food Cures: The Amazing Stores of 11 People
Who Beat Disease Using Raw & Whole Foods

Jerrod and Nikki are living examples of how great life can be when we eat to live. It is an honor to know that some of the recipes I created are among their favorites. If you are ready to be inspired for life, then this book is a must read.

Sarma Melngailis
Author, Living Raw Food and Raw Food, Real World

When I met Jerrod and Nikki back in 2003 our families spent a delightful afternoon together. Since then we have remained in contact and periodically gotten together. What Jerrod most reminds me of is "hope." He has always struck me as a "find-a-way" kind of guy. And he's always trying to pass along the hope that he has to others. Too many of us give up our dreams and settle for a lot less than God envisioned for us. Let Jerrod inspire you, instruct you, and make your hope come alive again.

Michael Donaldson
Director of Research, Hallelujah Acres

The Sesslers are an inspiration to many through their living example of tenacity, faith and real life. I have had the pleasure of teaching Nikki and Farrell when they were enrolled in my Certified Raw Food Chef course, after which they expressed their new found freedom and joy in the kitchen. This family is generous to share their story while kindly guiding us past the mind numbing maize of chaotic and sometimes untruthful information available. Reading Jerrod's health handbook, Five Percent Chance, will save you time and energy and guide you toward tangible changes that you can joyfully direct.

Mia Dalene, M.A.
Raw Food Chef, Author, Speaker & Traumatic Brain Injury
Survivor

I first met Jerrod when I called upon him as a salesperson in 2004. Although he purchased my product, he ended up giving me something much more valuable--he shared the story of his personal victory over cancer. At first I was skeptical (as I assume most people are) that the standard American diet is as toxic as it is. Admittedly, it took me several years of wrestling with the truth before I began to make significant changes in the foods I chose to eat. I could not have predicted the overwhelmingly positive impact that the consumption of raw vegetables and fruits has had on my health and the health of my family members. I personally challenge you to temporarily set aside what you think you know about nutrition and health while you read this book and read with an open mind. I encourage you to ask genuine questions, actively look for answers, and insist on finding the truth.

Chris Inverso – Tacoma, Washington
Speaker, Author, Coach. (www.ChrisInverso.com)

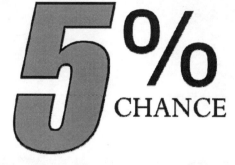

FIVE PERCENT CHANCE

5% CHANCE

Winning The *Cancer* Race

JERROD SESSLER
and NIKKI SESSLER

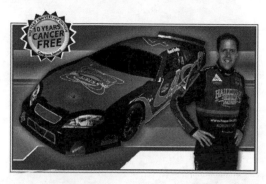

FIVE PERCENT CHANCE

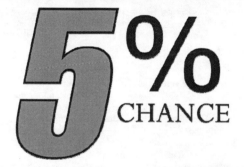

5%
CHANCE

Winning The *Cancer* Race

ToDoBlue
PRESS

SEATTLE, WASHINGTON

ISBN 978-0-615-33332-8

LCCN 2009940675

Published by ToDoBlue Press
206-763-6800

Edited by Hanne Moon, Lauren Bombardier, and Amy Michelle Wiley of Thru His Grace Writing & Editing Services, LLC.
Layout design by Diane Morton
Cover design by Justin Gingerella
Author photos by Joe Brockert

Printed in the United States of America
For Worldwide Distribution

DEDICATION

To my wife and kids for living healthy with me.

To those that choose a healthy lifestyle because it is right and not like me out of motivation to live.

To my friends at Hallelujah Acres who work tirelessly to spread the truth.

To everyone who has encouraged me along this challenging path.

CONTENTS

	Foreword	v
	Introduction	vii
Chapter 1	YCDI – You Can Do It!	1
Chapter 2	Racing Cancer for the WIN!	6
Chapter 3	Rejected For Dead	18
Chapter 4	Cancer, Heart Disease, Diabetes, Osteoporosis, etc.	29
Chapter 5	Focus Until It Feels Good	34
Chapter 6	What is the Hallelujah Diet?	39
Chapter 7	A Hallelujah Day	46
Chapter 8	Steer Clear to Win	54
Chapter 9	Supplements and Complements	60
Chapter 10	Hallelujah Acres Mission	67
Chapter 11	Living In Community	74
Chapter 12	Lighten Up!	78
Chapter 13	Q&A With Nikki	88
Chapter 14	Creation Foundation	101
Chapter 15	Fasting & Feasting	121
Chapter 16	The Facts	125
Chapter 17	Twisted Truth	131
Chapter 18	Life On The Go	139
Chapter 19	Simple Next Steps!	142
Chapter 20	Frequently Asked Questions	147
Chapter 21	Recommended Learning Tools	173
	Appendix A – Cancer Timeline	189
	Author Biography	204

Foreword

Jerrod Sessler has been a devoted personal friend, as well as a friend of Hallelujah Acres, for nearly a decade. We both share a passion not only for The Hallelujah Diet® but also for our Lord and Savior Jesus Christ. Jerrod and his wife, Nikki, have been on a journey of sharing the good news of the gospel of salvation and the message of health and healing that can only be achieved by nourishing the body according to the principles found in the Bible in Genesis 1:29.

In the year 1999, Jerrod's dreams were crushed when he was diagnosed with stage four metastasized melanoma cancer. He was given little hope of surviving beyond a few more years with the best that medicine had to offer. Because the doctors had so little to offer him, Jerrod turned to the Hallelujah Diet and Lifestyle, to which he had been exposed a few years earlier.

The Hallelujah Diet and Lifestyle® worked so well for Jerrod the doctors could no longer find any evidence of the cancer they said would take his life. Since his recovery, he has verbally shared his story with others in an effort to encourage them. Now you have the opportunity of reading about the remarkable journey God has lead him through as he shares his battles and victories in *Five Percent Chance*.

Jerrod is a man passionate about life and helping others. You will find his journey to be one filled with challenges as well as struggles and victories. In the pages of his book you will learn the causes of chronic degenerative diseases that destroy dreams and health. You will learn how to nourish the marvelous body God has entrusted to you in such a way that the innate self-healing within can bring about self-healing in most situations. You will be encouraged no matter where you find yourself in the seasons of life. Allow Jerrod to lead you on a pathway from where you are to a level of health you may find difficult to imagine.

I have learned from decades of research and personal experience that health is not achieved by treating symptoms with chemotherapy or other drugs, surgery, or radiation. The body cannot be drugged, burned, or mutilated into health. True healing can only take place when the body is provided conditions that are conducive to healing. Jerrod and Nikki will lead you on a pathway to better health as they discuss their personal journey this past decade.

As the proud parents of children they were never expected to have, they have learned how to nourish and encourage them in ways of which few parents of today have any knowledge. In the pages of this book, you can gain the knowledge they have discovered.

Jerrod and Nikki became Hallelujah Acres Health Ministers in 2002 in order to be better equipped to share the message of health with others. They have sponsored seminars in different areas near their home in Seattle, Washington. They have taught classes and developed organic food-buying programs as they seek to support and encourage those they minister to. You, too, will be educated, challenged, and encouraged as you read about their personal journey to the excellent health they are experiencing today.

— Rev. George Malkmus Lit.D., Founder of Hallelujah Acres

Introduction

I'm excited to be able to share my story with you, but more excited to know this will encourage you to look more closely at your own winning story!

The purpose of this book is to celebrate living through what could have been a death sentence and to share the things I've learned. For over a decade, I've passionately endeavored to learn the truths about healthy living. If you are also searching for answers, I know you will find the contents of this book encouraging and enlightening.

My vision for taking on this writing comes from my desire to encourage those who are facing health challenges, specifically those who may have recently been told they have no reason for hope, given their prognosis. My story and the facts I have amassed prove to me we have strong reason to maintain hope. The second group of people for whom I took on this project are for those who trust in God as their ultimate source of sustenance and foundation for their lives. I believe this message is for them. Ultimately, my hope is that this book brings encouragement to everyone who reads it.

Consider this your personal health handbook. *The Health Handbook* was the original title but *Five Percent Chance* sounded much more interesting and it connects with my prognosis. Doctors told me I had a five percent chance of still being alive ten years after the diagnosis. That was in 1999. Based on some quick math, my story is either a gross anomaly or I have learned some things that stacked the odds in my favor.

As I tell you my story, I want to share several basic truths I've discovered throughout this journey (I've also provided a chronology of my personal story in the appendix). I want our collective investment of time and resources (me to write and learn and you to read and learn) to yield healthy changes in your life. I'd like you to think of me as your virtual health coach—here to provide leadership, structure, guidance, instruction, examples, options and encouragement.

I realize that God can and does heal miraculously, but He more often than not chooses to let us use the resources He provides. I have been to many funerals throughout the years for people who prayed and waited instead of prayed and acted. One of my favorite books of the Bible is James because it's all about action.

So pray, and then act in faith!

CHAPTER ONE

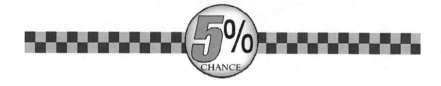

YCDI – You Can Do It!

It pains me to think of the thousands of people who walk out of doctors' offices and clinics each day, devoid of hope because of their circumstances and what standard protocol has to offer. It breaks my heart to know there are young mothers diagnosed with breast cancer who are being forced to consider the options for their soon-to-be widowed partners and beautiful children. It is a sad picture but unfortunately, these stories and more like this are being played out every day.

Education can come in the form of several options. We can take classes at the local community college, enroll in on-line curriculums, watch videos or visit our local library and book store. I personally find great comfort and solace in the rich mahogany wood of the library, with the tall shelves, comfortable chairs and spines of educational opportunities displayed before me.

How do you sift through the hundreds of books in the health section of the library or book store? To support and guide your enlightenment in this area, I have provided a list of recommended reading and educational materials in this handbook. Once you get a taste of what I'm going to share, I hope you'll want to dig in and learn more. There is a sea of misinformation out there and it's important that you have a solid foundation of knowledge upon which to make future decisions. For example, people that work in the field of counterfeiting are experts at identifying illegally produced money. They can spot counterfeit money because they spend an inordinate amount of time studying the real thing. Once they know the real deal like the back of their hand, they can spot a counterfeit quickly and easily. After working through this material, you'll be able to determine truth from fiction on your own.

During my visits to book stores, I often get a spike of excitement when I see a new cover, name, face, or author. The problem for many of us is that we don't know what the motivation is for all these publications. Sadly, most are not as scientific or noble as they lure us to believe. Today, I can flip through these books and quickly determine if they're based on any truth or if they're just more of the same rhetoric that clutters our culture, billboards, advertisements and, in turn, our minds. We'll look at some basics that will enable you to easily scan these resources and become proficient at determining fact or fiction.

I will cover a variety of topics so you can reference and use this handbook as a guide through your own journey to your best health. None of the subjects I cover in this book are exhaustive, so I've provided a variety of educational references where you can dive deeper into the topics that are of greater interest to you. Although I am a huge fan of on-going reading and education of all kinds, I don't believe you need to spend ten years learning as I have.

I would like you to let me help you over that educational hump, and share with you what I've learned. You can use what you glean from my experiences, as well as what you get from other sources, to tailor-make a program that meets your needs and brings you optimal results.

Don't rely just on what other people tell you, however. You need to test things out for yourself. You live in the greatest laboratory you could ever ask for—your own body! A good friend and health advocate references his "brain meter" and his body as a "laboratory of one." This does not mean there is a totally different solution for everyone, similar to what certain diets would espouse. What it does mean is that we are all in a different place with differing needs, and we must work with ourselves to grow to a healthy, vibrant existence.

Over the years, many people have asked me about the sufficiency and integrity of Hallelujah Acres. I discuss this more later in the book, but suffice it to say that I don't know it all, never will, and thus, have had to put a lot of trust along the way in Hallelujah Acres and others. You will need to make some serious decisions about who and what to trust. Our culture will point you to a standard medical doctor (allopathic practitioners) and although they have their place, they don't stand out as boldly or as singularly as many would have you to believe. In other words, they only know what they know. Like many of us, they've learned from their high school or college teachers and professors, books they've read, and experiences they have been through. Part of their problem is that practicing medicine is their means of survival, that is, how they feed their families, live their dreams, and so on. These doctors are not presented with many opportunities to get first-hand experience with using non-allopathic approaches to physical problems. I will introduce you to some doctors that have traversed this rough road of opposing the standard protocol.

As you continue through the educational process of learning the truth about your health, the full impact of your diet and lifestyle choices on your physical, spiritual and mental health will become more and more apparent. This process will force you to reconsider many of the habits and traits that you have picked up through your life from family, friends or other circumstances where you invested a portion of yourself. I hope that as you do this, you will see the necessary changes you need to make are like a child learning to walk. You start with a step, walk a few feet of steps, yards of steps, and then a mile of steps—taking pleasure in the results as you journey.

Yesterday, I was enjoying a nice lunch at a local salad bar with our kids. Someone who knows our story saw us eating at this particular restaurant and came in. This man's wife is suffering from a number of physical ailments including, but not limited to: cancer, weight control, and mental instability. Her illnesses are warping her spiritual perspective, and their marriage is threatened by the weight of the physical and spiritual battles being waged in their family. After he said "hi" to my kids, we stepped away to talk briefly. His features were set as he flatly stated, "This lifestyle change simply isn't going to work for us—it is simply too difficult and my wife is just not interested." This was shocking to hear for me because my perspective is different. I understand more fully now the ramifications of such a decision.

The changes that I and many others suggest are not hard and fast rules. It's not as simple as comparing it to driving north instead of south, using a red pen instead of a black one, or living on the east coast instead of the west coast. That's just not the way it is.

We need to be careful to avoid looking at changes or variations in our diet or lifestyle as an all-or-nothing thing. It is a journey, a stairway without an end. It is much like a dimmer switch that controls some lights. A little turn and the lights come on. A bit more turning and the lights get brighter. A standard light switch simply turns the lights on and off all at once. It is, unfortunately, the way many people see their lifestyle choices when in fact we live, and will continue to live, in a variable world. Our world requires us to consider each of our choices on a moment-by-moment basis. We must also realize that it is necessary for us to rely on a faithful God and not our past choices, our experiences, our successes or what we may call "decisions of permanence" because such things simply will not save us. Grace, received on a moment by moment basis, does.

The big challenge with the all-or-nothing perspective is that it is totally false and even prideful at its core. If you view diet and lifestyle as an all-or-nothing choice then you will never successfully allow yourself to make incremental changes or improvements. You are saying that you need to be perfect or you will not participate. There is folly in the search for perfection. I'm an idealist so trust me, I deal with this in myself all the time. What I am actually saying to God with my attempts at perfection is that I don't really need Him, or maybe more accurately, I don't want to need Him (because I know I really do). In reality, I don't have even a remote chance of achieving perfection. This is difficult for me, and for those around me, because I find it challenging to be satisfied with less than perfection. We will not start if we must start at perfection.

Let me encourage you to ask yourself what incremental changes can be made right now. You may only be able to grasp a very small percentage of the big changes that eventually need to happen. It may very well seem that the changes you do make feel bigger than they actually are. I remember the first few weeks feeling like I was having my world turned upside down. It felt like I was climbing a huge mountain. Later, as I continued to learn more, I realized that the changes weren't nearly as big of an obstacle as I first imagined them to be. As I got wiser in my choices, I could actually recognize where I had more opportunity for improvement.

We need to take steps in the right direction today, more tomorrow, and more each day afterward. The degree of success we have in mastering the choices that impact our daily, physical lives will be in direct relation to our quality and length of life. We may feel we're only achieving slight improvements if we measure our results against a perfect standard, but nothing we ever do will circumvent our need for that standard and, more importantly, our submission to that standard.

Remember, it's a climb. Climbing is challenging, but good in many ways. I will be here to help you along the way, as will many other people and great organizations such as Hallelujah Acres.

CHAPTER TWO

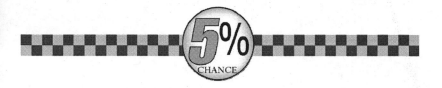

Racing Cancer for the WIN!

Some people ask me if my story is a miracle. What they are really asking is if I did the healing or if God did it through me. The answer is a resounding "yes!" God created us to live a certain way and He strengthened, provided and guided me to that path. I take no tangible credit for this although I was an active participant along the way. Your story can be a miracle too!

I am a deeply passionate man. I think on a grand scale and expect big things to happen. I rarely live "in the now" because I am normally planning the future. I choose to live in the now with my family, but I am disappointed if I don't anticipate or plan for everything else. For this reason, if for nothing else, you can understand why a terminal diagnosis at the age of twenty-nine was so shocking to me. I had already planned out the next couple of decades and I certainly didn't want to miss out on them. Little did I know I would indeed get to live long into the future, but my path didn't align at all with what I anticipated or planned prior to the diagnosis.

If we ever have the opportunity to meet, don't spend nearly as much time with me as you do with my wife, Nikki. She is one of the wonders of the world to me. I know of no one that she has disappointed upon meeting. She simply is a wonderful, incredible, beautiful, talented and loving person. Together, we have three great kids that I will talk a bit more about later. So you can see one of my treasures—my family. You may be surprised, however, to learn of the challenges even we have when it comes to eating to live.

There is a tendency in all of us in the western cultures to live to eat. Think about it. When was the last time you attended a social event that didn't involve food—most likely unhealthy food? Our gatherings seem to be an excuse to outdo each other, and most people scoff at the thought or consideration of healthiness in our choices. Food manufacturers and establishments have the upper hand by twisting our taste buds with flavor additives that are addictive and harmful. Everyone keeps raising the bar in terms of flavor excitement so we have in essence, as a culture, driven these companies to use more and more of these deadly, disease-creating additives. I will discuss these so-called "excitotoxins" in more depth as we move through our story. However, I'll warn you now that these flavor additives and processed foods are seated near the top of my hit list of things that cause great concern for our long-term health. The use of them is rampant and the results, in my opinion as well as those of others, are devastating.

While living in Seattle, Washington in 1998, Nikki and I began a journey that was founded in our mutual faith in a true and living God. We both quit our corporate jobs and started Hope4Youth, a non-profit organization dedicated to encouraging young people. We also started a little construction company. That was about the time that I began racing in one of the lower level NASCAR circuits.

My preferred sport is auto racing and I have been in pursuit of my racing dreams since I was a toddler. When I was only four, I told my mom that I wanted to drive racecars. I have always been competitive and loved speed. As a kid, I enjoyed bicycles, go-carts, motorcycles, and as I got older, full-sized NASCAR racecars.

Along with racing, another pursuit of mine is the illumination of truth. It's a never-ending chase trying to fully understand truth. This truth is the foundation for all ethics, beliefs, motives and wisdom. It never moves and is staying constant forever. It's the basis for my understanding of life, for understanding the world that we live in. I will never know everything there is to know, but education helps me continue to grow and understand.

It is a great honor to provide a place for truth to reside and to impact the world around me. It's a great honor to be alive and able to share with you the things that I have learned.

It is often hard to really believe that just a few years ago I was facing a very serious cancer diagnosis. Nikki and I were doing great. We were growing in our marriage, our business was flourishing, and we felt like our lives were having a positive impact in our community. Sometime during 1997, however, I noticed a mole on my back; it was itchy at times, discolored and irregularly shaped. I visited the doctor for a racing physical and he said not to worry about it, because it didn't seem like anything to be concerned over.

In late 1999, my mom, who was a nurse, grew tired of watching me back up against walls to scratch the mole. She scheduled an appointment with a dermatologist. One look and the mole was removed. Tissue samples that were sent for analysis revealed malignant melanoma cancer, and I quickly found myself at a specialized cancer care clinic with very little understanding of my options for healing.

At the clinic, they did a sentinel node biopsy—a test to determine where the cancer was exactly. They needed to know if it had metastasized or spread throughout my body. At age twenty-nine, sitting in the doctor's office with a lead ball in my stomach, I listened as I was diagnosed with advanced metastasized melanoma, a serious skin cancer that had already spread throughout my body by the lymph system. The doctors gave me a 5% chance of living past my thirties with no treatment, and up to a 20% chance of doing so with medical treatment. Neither of these options held a lot of promise.

A quick search on metastasized melanoma will reveal that it is a very serious form of cancer, contributing to around 2% of all cancer deaths annually. Metastatic melanoma in particular means that the cancer has spread, commonly via the lymph system, from the original location. To date, there is no known tracking mechanism other than inflamed (enlarged) lymph nodes or a tumor that is at least the size of a dime. Therefore, it is difficult for a patient to know if the cancer is gone or simply growing in the background until it reveals itself again. Melanoma tends to wreak even more havoc during a subsequent bout of it because it has had time to spread into multiple locations; it grows generally unnoticed until it is of significant size.

My discussions with oncologists centered on treatment options, including taking the drug Interferon, well known for its toxic side effects. I must mention here that one of the toxic side effects of Interferon is that about 5% of the people who take it actually die from the drug itself. Other slightly more palatable options included participating in a double-blind, two-year cancer study not knowing if I was receiving a sugar pill or the new experimental medication. Another option was chemotherapy, to achieve what one doctor called a "clean sweep of your system." The whole "clean sweep" terminology really tipped me over. It doesn't sound so odd now, and I guess it got their point across, but it certainly didn't help me to agree to the treatment or feel any more comfortable about their true understanding of what we were fighting. The doctors were quite abrupt when mentioning that Nikki and I would probably never have children, and that I was done racing.

With that, you have to understand a little bit more about Nikki and me. When Nikki was a little girl, she had dolls and dreamed of one day being the mother of her own wonderful little babies. She dressed them, cared for them and loved on them as she does with our beautiful children now. I don't think I need to dig any deeper into my dream box to demonstrate what "not ever racing again" meant to me. This was an earth-shattering and unacceptable life theme for us. The idea of taking these two passions from us was simply not an option for our futures, based on everything we had ever dreamed about.

Nikki and I had spent a day with my uncle and aunt in Chicago two years before, during the summer of 1997. The company and relationships were wonderful, but mostly we were more than perplexed about their eating habits and lifestyle. They were really dogmatic about what they ate and very inflexible. They stuck with raw produce, salads, juices, etc. They could not eat anything (so it seemed) and of course, at that time, we would eat just about anything. As we have grown, we have come to realize the gap was a combination of culture, age, wisdom and maturity.

As for their eating habits, my aunt had suffered with multiple sclerosis many years earlier but lived a healthy life while eating their weird diet. This day turned out to be providential for us because it was the day and experience we raced back to when I was diagnosed. We got a copy of the video titled How to Eliminate Sickness, (now called God's Ultimate Way to Health), by Rev. George Malkmus, Lit.D.. Our entire family and a small contingent of friends gathered around the television at my sister's home on Christmas Day in 1999 to watch this video, and the results deeply impacted and changed the course of our lives. In my case, it was like I had gone from sleeping very deeply under a tombstone to living an exciting, vibrant, world-changing life. We believe the message we heard resonated as truth and that we were blessed by the knowledge. We set out to learn what we could and change what we had to. And change we did.

> FIELD NOTES: George Malkmus is the Founder of Hallelujah Acres, a health ministry organization whose chief purpose is spreading the good news that "You Don't Have To Be Sick!" See: www.hacres.com.

Some of the doctors were willing to work with us on a monitored program which would identify if the cancer spread, returned, or grew in other regions. I visited a dermatologist, surgeon and received a CAT scan at regular intervals for two years.

FIELD NOTES: The oncologist made it clear, with an affronted tirade, that he wanted nothing to do with us. I feel bad that so many doctors do not actually understand how very simple the path to health and healing can be. I feel even worse that our culture trains us to hold these fallible doctors up on a pedestal which requires them to achieve results above the capabilities they in fact can actually achieve.

I would enjoy taking calls from doctors inquiring about the results of my self-treatment. If their sole purpose is assisting people to achieve health and healing, then their course would be different. Doctors would build relationships with their patients, understand them, and track with them as coaches as they traverse various ailments. Clearly not all doctors should be lumped into these categories, but the numbers point so resoundingly to these actions and attitudes that we must give way and recognize that doctors get up and go to work each day and collect a paycheck for their services much like the rest of us.

Within months of implementing The Hallelujah Diet®, the doctors were amazed that things looked so great and asked us what we were doing. After two years, I decided to discontinue the CAT scans due to their possible toxic side effects. Every time I went in there, I had to drink the nasty shake needed for the machine to see my insides as I passed through the scanner. I couldn't take just a little sip of it either. They had this super-sized cup that they kept topping off. I drank until I must have had a half gallon of the stuff inside me. I began to think about how closely we had learned to watch what we were putting into our bodies and how interesting it was that the doctors were not required to show me the ingredient list on this "shake."

As an aside, one of the editors of this book had to have a CAT scan recently, and because of allergies, she had to have the complete list of ingredients in the barium shake used for the CAT scan imaging. Imagine her surprise when even the doctors had no clue what the shake contained but still insisted it was safe for her to drink. After all, it was a medical thing! It had to be safe, right? After obtaining the ingredient list directly from the manufacturer, she found out it was full of excitotoxins. She insisted they use something else for the procedure. This shows what a little bit of education can mean for you in every day life. Learning is the key to taking control of your health.

In addition to drinking that horrible shake each time I went into the machine, they also injected a horrible clear substance into my blood. I found something quite interesting but not at all enjoyable as part of this injection. Within milliseconds after they started the injection, my rectum would literally feel like it was on fire. How on earth did that junk travel through my arm, into my heart and get pumped all the way down to my behind in milliseconds, and even more importantly, why did it feel like that? After a few of those, I just felt like whatever was going into me was worse than just keeping track of my own health by the way I felt and the signals from my body.

> FIELD NOTES: At the close of the book, I have provided all the nitty-gritty details and the entire chronology of the diagnosis and doctor visits.

As I transitioned my diet and lifestyle, I began to really get more in touch with what my body liked and what it didn't like, and this knowledge really became helpful to me as I defined what I would ingest and what I would pass on. To this day, I use this same approach, which over time, becomes even more valuable. I could do a lot more damage more quickly to myself by eating unhealthy foods now than when my intestines were coated with a layer of fat, mucus, and bile. This layer somewhat shielded my organs from many of the toxins I used to eat but the overall lifestyle caused a myriad of other problems.

From the time we started, it took us about three months to clear out the food we had, and we struggled with what to do with many of the items. We gave some to the needy, threw a lot away, and ate the rest ourselves. I started drinking thirty-two ounces of carrot juice each day, and taking three tablespoons of a BarleyMax® powder, a whole food produced and sold through Hallelujah Acres. We immediately stopped eating all dairy and meat products and ate a lot of salads. In the first three months I lost forty pounds, and by the sixth year I was sitting at about sixty pounds under my previous weight. I was ironically close to what Dr. Fuhrman (author of Eat To Live) suggests is a healthy weight for a man my size. I feel better than I've ever felt in my life.

> FIELD NOTES: Like you, I really do enjoy food. I don't feel deprived EVER! Seriously, I really enjoy what I am eating and know that what I am eating is more satisfying and more fulfilling, not to mention healthier, than what anyone is eating on the standard western diet. To find out what I am eating today, search for me on Facebook or other locations on-line.

The blessings of living the Hallelujah lifestyle continue to this day. We now have three incredible Hallelujah kids—Gabe (2001), Farrell (2003) and Jake (2005). They all love fresh veggies and fruit, and want nothing to do with candy or other junk most kids their age crave. Each of them started getting BarleyMax® on their pacifier as young as three months. Each morning, I make a mix of BarleyMax®, BeetMax® and CarrotJuiceMax®. I like mine in water as a little juice starter for the day but all of the kids get a bit of each on a spoon (in the order listed) and they love it.

In general, none of the children have ever been sick or required drugs. Gabe overate on some vegan waffles in February of 2005 and that was our first "up at night" experience for our family. They have all had at least one overeating experience similar to this by now. It is simply their body refusing the junk they put in it or even just too much of a good thing. Sure, they have fallen out of bed or wet the bed here and there, but for the most part, they have slept through the night from a couple months of age. I mention this because I think our diet and their "levelness" plays a huge role in the overall success and stability of our family. I can't imagine the stress and strain of sickness in children and all the implications of that including, but not limited to, being up at night, fatigue (for Nikki and/or I as well as the kids), bad attitudes, and unclear thinking.

> FIELD NOTES: When we mix the BarleyMax®, CarrotJuiceMax® and BeetMax® in the mornings, we

generally use the following proportions to make our concoction: 5 parts, 2 parts, and 1 part respectively. I drink it in about 10 oz of water, Nikki uses just BarleyMax® in about 4 oz of water and the kids just eat the three dry right off a spoon.

Nikki and I attended Hallelujah Acres' Health Ministers training in Sacramento, California, during the late summer of 2002. The training is focused on educating people like us who desire to learn more about living a healthy, biblically-founded diet and lifestyle, and who have the desire to help others do the same. We currently teach seminars and food-preparation classes regularly. I love to share my passion and, unlike my wife, I also enjoy public speaking on topics for which I have great passion. Nikki is really interesting to listen to, however, and if someone really wants to hear her, she will speak as well. Because of this, I began to take on speaking engagements on the subjects of health and business ethics and of course, some racing stories get sprinkled into the mix. We launched the Hope4Health Foundation to support the Hallelujah Acres health ministry.

One of the tools we developed in conjunction with Hallelujah Acres is available on our web site at www.hope4health.org. This tool allows you to measure your health potential by answering a few simple questions. To do so, click on "Take the PerforMax Challenge." We launched an organic produce delivery service called Freggies (www.freggies.com) in 2006. The purpose of Freggies is chiefly to get fresh, organic produce into the hands of as many people as possible at a good price, and secondly, to enable Hallelujah Acres health ministers and other health advocates to build relationships with people locally. I have a long term vision for planting "Health Cafés" through another venture called Good2Go Café (www.good2gocafe.com) as well. It is intended to be an outreach for the health message, but also a partial solution to the overwhelming health care issues that our culture is facing.

As the years passed by, we continued to look at every aspect of our lives for areas where we could make some gains health-wise. I began to look at our lives as if they were on a scale—one side was toxic intake and the other was nutritional intake. For example, if we drink tap water we are adding to both sides of the scale because there are toxins in the water, but of course, some benefit as well. So, it made sense to start drinking distilled water with liquid minerals added back to it. Another example is the soaps we use in our home. Everything from body soap to laundry soap and every kind of cleaner in between was reviewed. We set up an account with Melaleuca and have really enjoyed their products as well as many that Hallelujah Acres offers. We also purchased a very good quality air cleaner. I am still in awe at how clear the air is on a sunny day with the sun shining through a window or skylight. No more air floaties!

There are other things to think about, such as building products. Kids' play centers, fences, and outdoor furniture are often built with highly chemically-saturated building products which protect the wood and make it last longer but the chemicals are very toxic to the body. If you like the fancy foam mattresses and pillows that have become mainstream the last few years, be careful. We open ours and let it sit in the garage for at least a few days (preferably a few months) before we put it on our bed. That gives them a chance to air out some of the toxins left over from the manufacturing process.

> FIELD NOTES: Hallelujah Acres supports the Hallelujah Acres Foundation, which focuses on studying the current and changing environment that we live and work in. For years they recommended the use of distilled water as the next-best option to the water from fresh, raw, organic produce. Plants are the best water filters! They suck up water from the soil, along with minerals, and then use it to build whatever fruit they produce. Recently they discovered that adding back some live liquid minerals to the distilled water was good as it alkalized the water and added back some of the good minerals to the water.

One of the best things I have noticed about living this lifestyle is how much clearer I think. I just have a lot more mental clarity. All my relationships are better with my God and Savior, with my wife, and with my family members. Communication is better. I make better decisions and that impacts everything I do. I have been blessed to be able to use my position as a cancer survivor, leader, NASCAR driver, businessman, husband and father as a platform to help spread the good news of Jesus and wonderful results of implementing The Hallelujah Diet®.

One of the people I met after I began this journey was Bill. Bill was in his late fifties and had contracted hepatitis C about twenty-five years prior. He had struggled with poor results from the various approaches and modalities of the medical community for many years. Finally one day, he heard that changing his lifestyle could have an effect on the hepatitis C symptoms. The lifestyle changes he learned were similar in nature to those taught by Hallelujah Acres. After just a few weeks, he experienced amazing results, so much so that he found himself riddled with fear. To Bill, it was just too much of a good thing. This may seem like an odd reaction, but it was quite true and real for Bill. He had achieved a level of mental clarity that he had never felt before and the experience was possibly like some sort of mental high.

He found that he could increase this feeling by the way he ate and by how much fresh juice he drank, along with other diet changes. He found that the full level of clarity was too much for him to be comfortable with, so he backed it down with cooked foods or pasteurized juices rather than raw or fresh juice. I would agree that there is a mental fog that seems to lift when I eat healthfully, but I never experienced a fear from the clarity like Bill did. I believe my personality thrives on such clarity while others may be overwhelmed or even desire a bit of ambiguity. I further wonder how much our spiritual lives play into this. Maybe Bill was seeing things that he had just not ever been taught to understand.

I am grateful for the growing relationship I have with many people at Hallelujah Acres and our extended family of people that we have met, helped, been helped by, and just generally been blessed to be associated with. At the Hallelujah Acres headquarters, there are people I know that truly live their mission. I believe Rev. Malkmus defines the word consistency with his message about how to get healthy. The leadership team at

Hallelujah Acres trusts in God to make it all happen, and they will do whatever it takes to help people understand how to become healthy and how to stay that way.

Because Hallelujah Acres is mainly a teaching ministry, all of us who are associated with it have an uphill battle to overcome the passivity and apathy towards on-going education. For some reason in our culture, interest in education is just not common. Our culture is filled with people who want to consume the moment without a care for the future. Most of us are more concerned about our status in society than the number of days we will actually get to enjoy that status. Unhealthy meals entertain us for the moment, but when culminated cost us up to 50% of our life. Knowing this, then do they really taste that good? Life generally begins to shut down or at least show significant downward trends at the age of fifty. Sure many people exist beyond that age but are they really living? They are limited in their activities due to their physical ailments or due to their prescribed drug regime. More on this later, but for now let me just make one final point.

Have you ever considered how you learn? I know that I enjoy learning by doing. As I have gotten older, I find that I also enjoy reading books and filling my days with meaningful thought and consideration of concepts I don't fully understand. How do you learn? It is disappointing to me that we don't appoint more time to education. We see K-12 as the requirement, rather than the prerequisite, to a life of learning. I believe our elementary years are simply a time for us to learn the basics and to understand how we learn individually. It is likely that those of you who are reading this book think in similar terms because you have taken the time to open this book, so maybe you agree that education should be an honor, even a blessing.

I believe in you. I know you can do anything with your life that you set out to do. If you are faced with a situation like I was or you have other issues going on, consider what you have learned here, and what preconceived ideas you may have due to misinformation you have adopted.

CHAPTER THREE

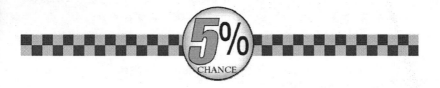

Rejected for Dead

It has not been a complete bed of colorful spring roses since my diagnosis. It has been great, but we have also made some mistakes and faced some challenges. The biggest one for me was dehydration the first couple of years.

It took me a long time to get to the point where I was eating 80% or more of raw foods, and during that time and probably years before, I had been dehydrating myself. A couple of times it was noticeably worse. On one occasion, I was scheduled for a speaking engagement about an hour from our home and I was suddenly in a terrible condition. I was tired, weak, had a headache and was very thirsty. I had only two hours before I was supposed to be on stage. We recognized the problem and I quickly started hydrating myself. I drank more than forty ounces of water before and during the drive to the event, and as soon as I got there I found a cool place inside to lie down. After about twenty minutes, I was due to speak. I got up, feeling fine, and did my thing. It was good that I was so well hydrated because the presentation was on an outdoor stage in the sun. I was soaking wet and felt wonderful within the first few minutes!

> FIELD NOTES: I eat over 95% raw now, so the hydration is not an issue with me any longer, but it is really important to find a healthy balance in your hydration. I rarely drink any water at all. This is only possible because I eat and drink so much water through my raw food consumption.

Deadly Toxins

During the first two years, we ate a lot of what we called "transitional foods." These were generally foods that were vegan (100% free of animal products, including dairy), but cooked. An example that I will use is a taco called a "Vegan" that is served at a local Mexican food bar. I ate there regularly during those first couple of years. Remember, I mentioned earlier that I started using my body as my barometer for determining what felt good and what didn't as far as the food I ate. After a while, I started to notice I didn't feel well after eating one of the vegan burritos the restaurant made. At first I thought it was because they were so enormous and I just needed to eat half, but I did some research and soon realized the problem was actually chemicals in my food— specifically monosodium glutamate (MSG). This particular company, like many fast food establishments, does not actually cook any of their food in the restaurant. It is processed in a huge food factory.

Rules for manufactured food: (per Jerrod)

> *Rule#1*: It can't cause immediate death.
> *Rule#2*: It must create profits!

Summary: If immediate death can be avoided then put all remaining emphasis on product profitability.

Is it just me, or does the thought of eating a lunch that was made in a factory seem wrong? Not the lunch room of a factory, but a factory that is specifically built to process and create food for us. My background is in manufacturing engineering, so thinking about factories and building things is not unusual for me. Have you ever considered where your food was made? There is a show on a cable network called "How It's Made" that often shows some of these food factory settings. One episode I watched recently with my kids showed how hot dogs were made. The audible response from them was comical and wonderful at the same time!

They showed a very large stainless steel mixing bowl of sorts. It was literally about the size of a small dump truck. That wasn't so bad, but watching them pour huge lumps of animal parts and pieces jammed together with fat and dripping with blood about did the kids in.

The bowl was, of course, some sort of mixing machine. This was the initial stage of combining the proper ingredients to make the desired type of hot dogs. The mix was then fed into a grinding machine, which eliminated any tiny animal body parts from surviving intact. Next, they showed how they stretch out the cow guts (intestinal sleeve-like pieces) to create the outer casing that will hold the mix together while it cooks. This was the fun part for the kids, because the goop shot out of the end of a machine into the sleeve-like intestine at a rate of about 1000 dogs per minute. They slowed the camera shot down so we could really see what was happening. After that, the dogs were cooked, the sleeve was sliced off, and the cooked hot dog-shaped slop headed to the packaging area. They also showed a similar mix used to fill up bread-shaped pans before cooking. These loaves were used for sliced sandwich meat. No wonder I became a big fan of mustard.

I have a large picture frame in my office that has a piece of white paper in it instead of artwork. On it, I write things that seem significant to me, things that seem to be almost revelation. One of the things I drew on it was a box about the size of the palm of my hand

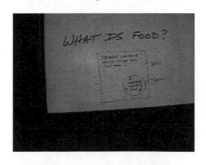

(about three inches). Inside the box I drew a small circle about the size of my fingertip. The three inch box represents what we choose to label as food, while the fingertip circle represents what actually is nourishing food or real food. The point is, we tend to feel comfortable eating stuff that is packaged in an appealing way by a worker in a factory. Does anything seem wrong with this? One of the books and movies I recommend is titled Fast Food Nation. In it you will learn about the machine and business end of food manufacturing. If a company's primary purpose is profitability, then how much concern are they really going to take in ensuring the food they create is good for you? Furthermore, if God created all the food we need in nature, then are we not playing god by attempting to modify or create new food? As soon as these companies can create their own species, then I will fully recognize their authority to also begin creating food for that species.

Food made in a factory is filled with chemicals to make it taste good after all the life is cooked out of it. It arrives in the restaurants in big plastic bags and is either microwaved or steamed to temperature. This food comes off the assembly line flavorless because cooking removes the majority of the flavor. Flavor additives are then added back into the food during and after cooking.

FIELD NOTES: I was interested in looking at the ingredients for a can of Campbell's Cream of Mushroom soup. I did a bit of research on-line and quickly realized that they do not share their ingredients on-line. I even emailed their customer support and was told I needed to visit a store and actually look at the label.

Give me a break. They can chant all they want about secret, company-owned recipes, but it is a bunch of marketing bunk. A six-year-old with a well stocked kitchen and a little help could replicate and possibly even improve upon any of their products in a couple hours. They are not hiding anything other than the fact that they are using massive amounts of excitotoxins in their food. Excitotoxins began with the additive called monosodium glutamate, or MSG. Because MSG itself has to be listed on the ingredients list of all manufactured foods, it is now sold under more than one hundred different disguised names such as hydrolyzed protein, sodium caseinate, yeast extract, textured protein and many others. Additionally L-cysteine, aspartate, and aspartame are excitotoxins that are not required by the FDA to be shown on food labeling. As if that wasn't bad enough, names like natural flavoring, bouillon, seasoning, malt extract, spices, carrageenan, enzymes, and many more are often hiding places for manufacturers to include excitotoxins in the foods they produce. In other words, the food manufacturers want to make it as difficult as possible for the finger to be pointed at them for using these substances in their foods. They know the dangers and they use them anyway. If they were ever to be questioned, as they should be, they would not have any excuse for their actions.

So what is the big deal with an excitotoxin and why should we be so concerned about them? According to Dr. Russell L. Blaylock in his book Excitotoxins, these are a group of excitatory amino acids that can cause sensitive neurons to die. Some of these compounds are found in nature and some are created artificially, such as kainate. When a neuron is exposed to a massive dose of MSG, the cell immediately begins to swell and dies within one hour. When a lower dose of MSG is used, nothing appears to happen immediately, but after the second hour the neuron suddenly undergoes rapid death.

I had the displeasure of experiencing two very unfortunate incidents of chemical poisoning, and both occurred just after eating at Mexican restaurants. One was after a meal at one of the locations of a fast, casual Mexican food chain in Seattle and the other was just after a meal at a local Mexican restaurant in Eagle, Idaho. Both experiences turned out to be two of the most uncomfortable, painful situations I can remember and brought me closer to death than the cancer did. During a family vacation, we had to extend our time at a lake in McCall, Idaho, because I was in bed for about thirty-six hours, and I wasn't sure if I was going to live. I couldn't eat anything and all I could drink was water. I was chemically poisoned and in a lot of pain. I could not sleep for more than an hour or two at a time and I just hurt all over. Chemical poisoning is very different than congestion or a virus or similar types of illnesses. It comes quickly, hurts a lot, has to be flushed out, and then leaves rather swiftly. After a couple of days of struggling in pain, drinking water, and lying in bed, it finally passed and I was up and about and feeling fine. The reaction to a meal at the local fast, casual Mexican joint was less severe.

Rejection

During that period of weeks and months after my cancer diagnosis, I remember thinking I should get a t-shirt saying, "Why are you treating me like I am going to die soon?" It was amazing how people wrote me off. There is something about having a terminal illness that makes others want to disassociate themselves from you (or so they think). Fortunately I am married to my wonderful wife, Nikki, and she would never have anything to do with such a callous response to people's fears and feelings (so I never got the t-shirt). I have talked with other survivors though, and this does seem to be a common response from the people around them. I can remember when I associated "cancer" with "death" almost as directly as I associated "fast" to "racing"! When I hear of someone with a diagnosis of cancer now, I get excited because I realize there is a cure. People who receive a cancer diagnosis are most likely going to have the motivation necessary to make some serious changes.

Yes, it is exciting…when they listen.

As I talk with others who have had a terminal or near-terminal diagnosis, I find we all share a common experience in the way we felt about the human reaction to impending death. The initial reaction is shock. Some people desire to help, but most seek the answer to the inevitable question, why? Romans 12:2 indicates that if we want to know the will of God for our lives through testing and approval, then we must first be transformed. How? By the renewal of our minds. *"Do not be conformed to this world, but be transformed by the renewal of your mind, that by testing you may discern what is the will of God, what is good and acceptable and perfect."* (ESV)

Well, I certainly want to know God's will for my life, so how do I renew my mind? I mention this scripture here not because I intend to fully answer the question of how we change, but because I want to demonstrate that it's futile to ask the "why" question of God every time things don't go as we plan. We are much better served by getting to know His plan for us and how we fit into His great story.

After the initial shock, others have confirmed with me that friends, family, and coworkers just sort of drift away. The relationships begin to die because the people think we are going to die. It is easier for them to create some physical separation so when the day comes that they hear our life has ended, the pain will be somewhat mitigated.

For those like me who live through the diagnosis, the more human reaction becomes bizarre. People act as if nothing ever happened. I think this took about five years for me. With some people, it is still uncomfortable when we see each other. I know you are probably thinking, "Isn't that what you want, for people to treat you normally?" Well, yes and no. I want people to treat me normally just as all of us do, but I also want people to recognize that God did a miracle through me, and He wants to do one through you as well.

Maybe you don't have cancer or a severe physical problem at all. Maybe He wants to heal you in your marriage or your relationship with your family. It could be that He wants to work a miracle through mistakes you have made in your past that still hold you back today. The point is He wants the best for us, and it is ridiculous for us to look into the face of a beautiful scene, created by God, and ignore the fact that He, in His sovereignty, worked through a situation and that He deeply wants to do the same in all of us. All we need to do is be willing to participate, and to be active in seeking Him, so we know what our part in the process looks like.

Allergies

You can check with my mom, but I was literally the allergy prince as a kid. My eyes would swell shut if someone even mentioned the season of spring within fifty feet of me! I didn't get sick regularly, but I had my fair share along with viruses and other bugs.

In the years I have been doing this, I would estimate my allergy issues are over 90% better and often non-existent, but I do deal with them in minor ways occasionally. Sometimes I may need to do some refining in my diet, or I may need to get away from some sort of chemical or issue that is bothering my body. For instance, I got pink eye in 2006, which was sort of uncomfortable, but it looked much worse than it felt. I was told it was a virus and would be tough to avoid regardless of my health. I didn't visit the doctor for it and only took natural oils recommended by a friend. It was pretty amazing how quickly it passed. The oils, for reference, were oregano and rosemary. Don't ask me how they worked, but I can tell you that there is more about essential oils that I need to learn in the coming years.

We need to approach allergies with our eyes wide open because that is an area where we can easily be deceived. I began to learn about this a few years ago when someone told me that they were allergic to a food I felt that, by design, they should not be allergic to. The food was spinach, but that doesn't really matter because I have heard people say this about all different types of food. Nuts and grains tend to be the most common, and there may actually be some validity to their claims with these because most nuts and grains are processed. So, the question is, are we allergic to the food item, or to the processing, including possible added substances? Even with produce, could it be that we are actually allergic to the pesticides that are used to speed the growth, size and perfection of the produce? These solutions are what I consider the low hanging fruit. Unfortunately most of us respond to just these. There is however a deeper consideration.

Simply identifying the properties of the food or substance would be relatively simple. If we are allergic to spinach then we simply avoid spinach or maybe we look at what spinach is made up of to try to determine if there is some property of the spinach that is actually the culprit. Again, I believe this is the obvious response but it ignores the real issue. Our allergic reaction to many substances must be a symptom of a different problem.

An allergic reaction is defined as an over-reaction of our self-healing system, our immune defenses. For some reason, our internal army has been aroused to fight an enemy but in some cases, our protective army over-reacts against what should be considered harmless or possibly even helpful. It is important to recognize that this immune reaction is natural and a necessary function of our overall immune system but at times it explodes into an over-reaction.

Let me use an example. You walk out your front door and water drips on your head. The ground is wet and you know it's been raining. You happen to have had an elaborate gutter system installed on your house that is supposed to catch the water from the roof and divert it to downspouts and an alternate drainage system. You look at the gutters and assume they've failed to do their job. You try caulking the joints but still water is dripping on your head. You try putting diverters on the roof to funnel the water a different direction, but still water is dripping on your head. In all of your efforts to fix the gutters you failed to realize that gutters only capture some of the problem. Dripping gutters are a sign (symptom) that it is raining. The fact that it is raining is the source of the problem.

Likewise, we have created unpredictable environments within our bodies because of the toxins we ingest in our food and our breath. We can't flatly say we are allergic to this or that without a deeper consideration of the environment we have created in our bodies by our lifestyle choices. This is especially true if the things we are claiming to be allergic to are natural foods made by our Designer. If you get a headache after eating an orange or a rash after eating broccoli, then clearly there is another problem. That problem is not the orange or the broccoli. If you experience an allergic reaction after consuming something that should be nutritional and beneficial then there is a deeper problem inside the body, not inside the healthy food.

I have had multiple Crohn's patients tell me that they were told to avoid all greens due to some digestive issues that cause flare-ups within their digestive systems. What they are actually being told is to avoid fiber because the fiber is abrasive to the digestive system. This abrasiveness is irritating and uncomfortable to an already compromised digestive system. This scenario represents the very same thing I am saying about allergies. The very thing that all of us need as a primary piece of our diet is raw, leafy, dark greens. In the case of a Crohn's patient, they may need to juice these and attempt to avoid fiber as much as possible until they improve the condition internally. For allergies, we need to consider the overall health of our system, make changes to improve deficiencies and not get distracted along the way because what we know to be true doesn't seem to be working on an individual basis (i.e. everyone else can eat spinach but I must not be made to consume that).

Be skeptical of direct cause-and-effect lines drawn between any food and any allergic reaction. Realize that other factors inside your body contribute to the allergic reaction just as much, if not more, than what you actually ate. If I was allergic to some natural food that God clearly designed for us to enjoy, then I would look at the rest of my diet and overall toxic load (past and present) to try to determine what may be contributing to this reaction. I would make some changes and test again until the allergic symptoms disappeared. In other words, test for allergies and then change the condition in your body, not the reaction to food.

There are some things that we really are not designed to eat and will kill us instantly. Other things were clearly designed for us to ingest for our nourishment and benefit. It is interesting that we are smart enough to avoid the things that will kill us instantly, yet we choose to accept the consumption of those things that cause slow death.

My family generally lives free of allergies and sicknesses. We never have to clean out our noses or sinuses in the shower like I can remember doing in the past. I believe this pattern of health enables our family to live with less stress, fatigue and uncontrolled emotions. In other words, because of our lifestyle choices, life is just easier in our home than in many homes. We do have a wonderful family and an incredibly fun family life. This is in part possible due to our healthy diet choices.

CHAPTER FOUR

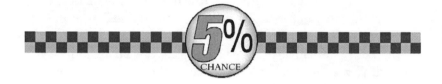

Cancer, Heart Disease, Diabetes, Osteoporosis, etc.

What causes disease?

Diseases are caused by toxins. You can also look at it as toxic load in excess of our physical ability to overcome. I have explained this in the past as an old-style balance scale. If the toxins are stacked up on the left then we need to pile the same amount of nutrition or immunity building blocks on the right. It really is that simple. Overcome the toxic load and you will completely avoid physical ailments.

> FIELD NOTES: We must understand that toxins can include things other than food. The air we breathe, clothes we wear and people we make contact with can all contribute to our toxic load. We can create a toxin load

through stress. This can lead to actual physical toxicity of our own making and mental or spiritual breakdown.

How is disease cured?

There are only two ways your body can be cured and neither one is a pill. There is no pill that has ever cured anything and suggesting that it does, could, or will someday is pure insanity. Pills mask symptoms, which is why we continue to take them. The issue or disease is not cured—it is hidden by the work of the pill. If it is possible, would it not be better to cure the problem rather than mask the symptoms?

The first method to being cured is the most common method by far. This is healing that takes place due to our built-in self-healing mechanisms. It is our responsibility to nourish our bodies in such a way that we enable these internal functions to operate properly. The second method for curing disease is much less commonly experienced—it purely by the grace of God working in and through us by the power of the Holy Spirit. It is an absolute possibility, but to our knowledge rarely enacted—at least not how we expect.

In my eyes, the two ways I am suggesting are one and the same. God created our physical bodies and He gave us responsibility over the care of these bodies. He also sustains us from moment to moment. A real, tangible way to look at this is by knowing that all physical power on earth comes from a single source of energy, the sun. Big corporations and even countries attempt to wield their control over power, but it is actually free to all of us and is new every day. Similarly, His power lives through each of us directly and is, by very nature, His and not ours. Therefore we are completely reliant upon Him and His perpetual grace even if we choose to deny it.

> Exodus 15:26 says, *"If you will diligently listen to the voice of the LORD your God, and do that which is right in His eyes, and give ear to His commandments and keep all His statutes, I will put none of the diseases on you that I put on the Egyptians, for I am the LORD, your healer."* (ESV)

Am I cursed because of my genes?

No. You may have some stronger predispositions towards a certain disease or ailment, but you are not cursed or destined to die of what ails your parents, grandparents, cousins, or other family members. The biggest consideration to evaluate when you are attempting to measure your risk of disease as it relates to the suffering of your relatives, is the amount in which your day-to-day routine or habits resemble theirs. In other words, the fact that you mimic the same behavior as your parents is more powerful than the fact that you got your genes from them when it comes to disease. Stop doing the bad things that they do and you will experience different results.

Another factor to consider when looking at your family history and lineage is generational degeneration. With each passing generation there is a building of physical brokenness. Someone that is unhealthy is going to pass on not only their unhealthy habits but also their physical ailments or propensities therein. This is exacerbated by the rapid decline in overall food quality in recent generations. What this looks like in practice is that people are getting diagnosed at younger ages and showing signs of general ailing sooner than previous generations. This plays out until we begin to experience infertility which in many cases is simply a physical response from the body refusing to conceive due to a build up of physical deficiencies. The body simple cannot produce offspring after repeated generational declines. This was proven in a ten year study by Dr. Pottenger which concluded in 1942 where he experimented with the effects of diet on groups of cats. He showed that after generational degeneration, the cats were unable to reproduce.

To learn more about the cause and cures for various ailments, Dr. Joel Fuhrman's book titled Eat to Live is probably the best overall resource I can recommend. Organizationally, Hallelujah Acres has a swath of amazing resources of which Eat To Live is just one. The China Study by Dr. T. Colin Campbell is another wonderful resource and is especially useful for analytical types (like me) who really want to understand some of the science and the data. The China Study is written well within the grasp of those of us who aren't doctors, so don't worry about getting in over your head. In it, Dr. Campbell discusses the diseases that are directly associated with western diets heavy in animal consumption while contrasting them with the diets of less advanced societies. If you want to cure yourself from ever being tempted to taste another bite of anything that came from an animal, then The China Study would certainly be worth a few hours of your time.

Ultimately, this struggle is mainly a mental one. You need to first educate yourself to know what is right, and then you have to stand guard and bash your habits in the face a few thousand times until you retrain your mind to what is good and right (Romans 12:2). The nice thing is that you can begin to experience wonderful results almost immediately with even some simple changes to your habits.

Pick Your Ailment. Pick Your Recipe.

If you desire one of the following types of ailments, then simply follow the respective recipe and you will be well on your way.

Long term debilitating disease.

If you have a deep desire to have an attractive nurse doting over your failing body while you lay in a hospital bed, suffering from complications because of a long term debilitating disease, then based on my experience and studies, you simply need to consume as much animal protein as possible. Animal protein, in any and all forms, will do the trick, including organically grown, grass fed, as well as the really nasty stuff filled with chemicals and growth hormones. Even dairy contains more than enough pus-filled animal protein to greatly assist in the damage of your God-made physical body. I will discuss the reasons why I don't believe we were intended to consume animals later in the book. Also, the section on recommended reading has numerous resources you can utilize to learn about this like I did.

Short term sickness, cold, flu or other illness.

If sickness is the frequent and standing excuse to miss work, school, church or anything else on your schedule, then based on my experience and studies, you would simply need to consume as much refined simple sugar in as many forms as possible. This can come in the form of sugary drinks, highly refined and processed foods or many other forms and sources of simple sugars.

Obesity.

I have a dear friend who once told me that she gained weight years prior because she didn't want to be constantly confronted by men with their plans and schemes. If you, too, would like to avoid being attractive to others or yourself, and you think the gluttony of food would be an easy remedy, then don't fear. The solution is at hand. Based on my experience and education, you can simply allow the majority of your diet to be processed and packaged foods. In so doing, you will bypass your body's natural ability to satiate the strongest of appetites once nutritional satisfaction is achieved. This will certainly do the trick, and before long you will be hydro-pressing your wardrobe from the inside out and be forced to the plus-size section of the department store. Better yet, you can just buy a bunch of sweats since they so easily stretch with a bulging body.

CHAPTER FIVE

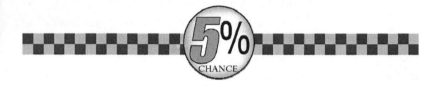

Focus Until It Feels Good

How many times have you heard stories of a couple struggling in their marriage that head off to a weekend seminar and come back revitalized, possibly even pregnant? Maybe this example isn't too distant for you. It certainly is a popular one, and on the surface it seems like a very good result. And, likely in some cases, the value that comes from such a weekend, or maybe pieces of it, contributes to an overall end result that is better than where they were before. Maybe it is a series of these seminars that builds up to a crescendo where something just clicks and he (or she) finally gets it.

As you read this, know that I am all for continuing education. In fact, I made a point of including a chapter on that very subject in this book. Also, I am not saying that we should avoid these weekend seminars and other types of on-going education. It's quite the opposite, in fact. If you take a look at my wife's and my schedule, we are proving it in our own lives.

For some of us however, we do need to adjust our perspective on why and how we go about these opportunities. More often than not the result is something like the following: A couple finds themselves in a point of their relationship a few months after the wedding when the bliss and newness of the marriage wears off. Now they have a chance to live together and they realize how annoying they each are. She snores at night and for some reason doesn't always look as put-together as she did on their dates. He seems a bit lazy and always seems to be chasing some prize—other than her. After all, she is won already, right? They have some friends who mention they are attending a seminar in a couple weeks, so this couple signs up as well.

The seminar comes and the education is amazing. The result is wonderful, and they actually feel higher after the weekend than they did on their honeymoon. What a difference some focus can make! They float in the clouds for a few days until signs of the same patterns that dragged them down previously begin to become apparent once again.

I call the weekend seminar "the spike" and the ensuing months "the slide." Not too many months later they find themselves in about the same place, if not a little lower, than they felt before. Now they have the burden of realizing that the seminar was a bit of a hot shot at best and that there are still severe problems. They insist it must have been the wrong seminar, so they sign up for another weekend seminar. Off they go successfully training themselves to live the spike and slide instead of actually growing.

This is not an uncommon scenario in our culture. What is the problem? Clearly that isn't the point of this book so let me give you the short version: apathy, laziness, lack of trust in God, false idols, desires that become expectations, men who simply don't understand themselves (seriously, woman are not the confusing ones), pride, arrogance, sin, folly, Satan, mistakes, false paradigms, and inaccurate world views.

The point of this section is that this couple, as well as anyone trying to lose weight, who succeeds in something such as overcoming an illness or stopping a habit, will face similar mental challenges as they adventure along. How will they respond to these challenges? How will this couple respond after seventeen weekend seminars with the same spike-and-slide results? Are they willing to face the facts of their situation? Are they over-optimistic about their circumstances? Will they give up?

In Jim Collins' best-selling book, *Good to Great*, he addresses this very issue head on. In this context, he and his research team apply this concept to leaders of various companies. How do they answer these questions as they relate to their businesses? The results are astounding, and the relationship between just being good and achieving greatness are inextricably connected. Collins dubs this "The Stockdale Paradox" where we are challenged to "retain faith that we will prevail in the end, regardless of the difficulties." At the same time, we are to "confront the most brutal facts of our current reality, whatever they might be."

So, it seems that successful people are those who can maintain a stoic focus on the end game, result, or goal while at the same time openly and honestly understanding where they stand. This is not to say that just because I might be three laps down with a mediocre racecar, doesn't mean I can't somehow come back to win the race. It simply means I need to stay focused on winning while at the same time understanding my situation. In a racing situation, this focus enables a team to make decisions they may not otherwise make, in order to earn back laps they otherwise would not have gained.

Admiral Jim Stockdale served in the United States Navy during the Vietnam War. He was a prisoner-of-war, was tortured and beaten without knowing when he would be released. Admiral Stockdale secretly led a group of prisoners through a mental journey that lasted eight years for him.

According to the account from Collins, the Admiral indicated the optimistic didn't make it. Those that set false targets such as this Christmas, Easter, or the next Thanksgiving would end up dying of a broken heart. Those that simply faced the fact that they did not have a date, but yet were somehow able to continue to believe they would, in fact, be vindicated, were the winners.

So what does all of this have to do with diet and lifestyle? Do you want to make a big change, only to slide back to where you are now—or worse? Or, do you want to invest heavily in education, make small changes and maintain a stoic focus on where you want to be five or ten, or even thirty-five years from now? Clearly, these are opposite directions and the results are going to be immeasurably different as well. It is the difference between a marriage and a date. Casually dating a healthy lifestyle isn't going to get you the results you want. Committed marriage, with a vision for what can be, presents your best chance for success.

Is there a more pervasive and controlling factor in our lives which reaches more people, touches more lives, and yields more respect? The only one I can come up with is God Himself. Clearly God is omnipotent and all-knowing. He is ever-present and amazing. I am not contesting any of that, however food is quite literally in a realm of its own I don't know if this is true in cultures outside of the west, be we westerners hold nothing more closely than our food. Some would say that sex or money vies for the position, but I would disagree simply because these don't impact as many people. Not everyone is greedy and most women simply don't have the sexual prowess of most men. There are some connections, however. If you step up one rung above these, you will find a couple of pernicious false idols standing tall— power and comfort. Food, sex, and money all feed comfort, while at the same time for some people, they also feed the power, control, and self-righteousness.

Food, however, impacts every one of us. It was even the tool Satan used to entrap Adam and Eve, and I believe he continues to use it today to taunt us and to lead us astray. A friend of mine recently helped me to see this more clearly. He said that the love of food is the only false idol you can't just knock down and walk away from. Sexual sin, gambling, laziness or addictions of any kind can simply be walked away from at any moment. One must simply make the choice to do so. In so doing, they are essentially saying that they choose God, the real Deity, over their false idol and if they choose Him, they need never revisit that false idol's temple again. What about gluttony (the love of food—to excess)? We still need the nourishment that comes from the food, so we need to continue to eat. We can't just kick it to the curb like the bottle. It is likely for this reason that it is so very difficult for people to openly see the reality of their relationship to their food.

For those of you who do finally achieve a glimpse of the master control that your food has on you, you can begin to apply the principals of the Stockdale Paradox successfully. You will begin to see the truth about your situation and the control that has been yielded to food. You will recognize the impact your food and lifestyle choices have on your existence. From there, you can begin to build hope that you can and will be able to achieve success in using food for fuel, and refocusing your life on eating to live rather than living to eat. Realizations like this are sobering and they remind me of sayings like "ignorance is bliss." Hopefully I have not ruined your bliss. Well, maybe I do hope that I have. I believe the challenges we face after bliss are purposed to take us to a greater joy.

So, you may ask, when will it start to feel as good as the title of the chapter suggests? Based on what we learned about the Stockdale Paradox, the answer to that is very likely going to be different for every person. If I told you so many days, weeks, months, or years, then that would be setting you up like one of the over-optimists. Not only that, but your situation is uniquely yours and by that very nature has a completely different set of circumstances. What I will promise you is that the path does get sweet, very sweet, and there are innumerable treasures in plain sight along the way that are left for you to enjoy.

CHAPTER SIX

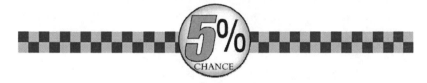

What Is The Hallelujah Diet®?

I have included some information from the Hallelujah Acres®
web site (www.hacres.com) in this chapter. After I present their
information I will reflect on it a bit and explain some nuances,
additions, and changes that my wife and I have made along the
journey. It is important to recognize that I fully support
Hallelujah Acres®, their teaching, and their leadership. This is
not because they are perfect, but because they know a lot more
than I do. They are focused on getting the very most out of our
physical bodies for the glory of God each day. Any question I
have had, they have answered many times over.

This does not mean I proceed blindly. Even though they have all
the answers, you and I have unique lives. We have circumstances
and situations that simply can't be lumped into some general
teaching for all. It is important to understand that there is one
perfect diet (conceptually) for all of us, but that there are nuances

according to our individual situations and circumstances that we need to consider as we make changes.

To begin with, one thing we need to look at is our willingness to accept and adopt change. If we aren't willing, then this could serve as a stumbling block to our success and may slow our progress as compared to someone who is making healthy changes. An example could be a person dealing with multiple physical problems, because the combination of their given situation may dictate different approaches. Someone who is obese and has cancer may approach the first year or two differently than someone who is obese with diabetes, or someone else that has Crohn's disease along with arthritis.

Here is the information from the Hallelujah Acres® web site. I would encourage you to get on their mailing list to receive information from them, such as publications, newsletters, and health tips. They have a wealth of knowledge, and they have nothing but your best in mind.

> Hallelujah Acres® is a Christian ministry that provides education, products, services, and other resources to help people everywhere understand and practice God's ways to ultimate health.

> The Hallelujah Diet & Lifestyle® is whole-person health at its God-given best. When you feed your body the nutrients it needs through The Hallelujah Diet®, and nurture your mind and spirit through the Hallelujah Diet & Lifestyle®, every part of you will know and experience the optimal health we were all meant to have.

The Hallelujah Diet & Lifestyle® is biblically, scientifically, and personally validated. The biblical foundation is found in Genesis 1:29 and is covered in more detail elsewhere in this handbook. As if the Bible isn't enough, scientific evidence is well substantiated by hundreds of studies as well as research performed by non-biased doctors, scientists, and other organizations. To learn more about some of these, see the book recommendation section in this handbook. For personal evidence, I am living proof that the Hallelujah Acres Diet & Lifestyle® works and is founded in fundamental and basic truth. Many people are encouraged by my testimony and many have adopted all or part of the Hallelujah Diet & Lifestyle® thanks to the story that God has birthed through me. It is an honor to know that my personal experiences have helped encourage others.

In short, the Hallelujah Diet® is a mix of part raw or living foods—meaning foods that have not been cooked and foods that are partly cooked. Regardless if the food is cooked or raw, the contents of the Hallelujah Diet® are always plant-based whole foods or food that comes from living foods at some point. You will learn in the next few pages what is or is not allowed within the guidelines of the Hallelujah Diet®. I want to remind you as you read this of the biblical, scientific, and personal validation because it is likely you are going to be searching for some of your staples or favorite foods and you are going to find them on the wrong side of the fence, so to speak. Just be patient and remember this is not an all-or-nothing sort of thing. My encouragement is to:

a) Maintain an open mind to change, realizing that what you have been taught previously may not have been truth.

b) Make small, incremental changes with stoic focus on long-term benefits and the eventual culmination of all your steps into a great big, wonderful result.

c) Never stop feeding your mind with good teachings from those you have a reason to trust.

Once you understand The Hallelujah Diet®, you will find that it is very simple to prepare and follow the ratio of 85% raw and 15% cooked food each day. So, let's dive right in.

The 85% Portion
This is the Hallelujah portion of The Hallelujah Diet®—an abundance of God's natural foods that are uncooked (raw) and unprocessed. The dense living nutrients found in raw foods and their juices are the things that meet and satisfy your cells' nutritional needs. When you eat these living foods, you will find you no longer have to deal with hunger pangs or cravings.

Live foods also produce abundant energy and vibrant health. The following are items from each food category that fit into the 85% portion of each day's food intake:

Beverages . Freshly extracted vegetable juices, BarleyMax®, CarrotJuiceMax™, BeetMax™, and distilled water with WaterMax™ added.

Dairy Alternatives . Fresh almond milk, creamy banana milk, as well as frozen banana, strawberry or blueberry "fruit creams."

Fruit . All fresh fruit, as well as unsulphured organic dried fruit (sulphur is often added as a preservative and should be avoided). Limit consumption to no more than 15% of daily food intake. (Fruit juice is included in this 15%, and is not recommended in large quantities).

Grains. Soaked oats, millet, raw muesli, dehydrated granola, dehydrated crackers, and raw ground flax seed.

Beans. Raw green beans, raw peas, sprouted garbanzo beans, sprouted lentils, and sprouted mung beans.

Nuts and Seeds . Raw almonds, sunflower seeds, macadamia nuts, walnuts, raw almond butter, or tahini (eat sparingly).

Oils and Fats . Extra virgin olive oil, Udo's Choice Perfected Oil Blend™, Udo's Choice DHA Oil Blend™, raw unrefined flax oil and avocados.

Seasonings. Fresh or dehydrated herbs, garlic, sweet onions, parsley, cayenne pepper and salt-free seasonings.

Soups . Raw soups

Sweets . Fresh or frozen, all fruit smoothies, raw fruit pies with nut/date crusts, date-nut squares, etc.

Vegetables . All raw vegetables.

The 15% Portion
The following cooked foods make up the 15% portion of The Hallelujah Diet®, and follow the raw salad at the evening meal. This portion can be very delicious, and actually proves beneficial for those trying to maintain body weight.

Beverages . Caffeine-free herbal teas and cereal-based coffee-like beverages, along with bottled organic juices.

Dairy . Non-dairy cheese, rice milk, and organic butter (use all sparingly).

Fruit . Stewed and unsweetened frozen fruits.

Grains . Whole-grain cereals, breads, muffins, pasta, brown rice, millet, etc.

Beans. Lima, aduki, black, kidney, navy, pinto, red and white beans.

Oils . Mayonnaise made from cold-pressed oils.

Seasonings . Light Gray Celtic® Sea Salt (use sparingly).

Soups . Soups made from scratch without fat, dairy, or table salt.

Sweeteners . Raw, unfiltered honey, rice syrup, unsulphured molasses, stevia, carob, pure maple syrup, date sugar (use very sparingly).

Vegetables. Steamed or wok-cooked fresh or frozen vegetables, baked white or sweet potatoes, squash, etc.

Response to the Hallelujah Diet® from Jerrod:

While this list may appear a bit limiting at first, there are hundreds, if not thousands, of exciting recipes that meet these criteria. I regularly have people comment there is simply no way they could eat as I do. The reality is that they are the ones who are living the limited lives. They only eat what they were brought up with or what the local eateries serve. These people generally visit just a handful of restaurants, and order the very same thing nearly every time. Combine that with the fact that they have only a few recipes at home that they make with any regularity, and then come back and tell me who has the variety and who doesn't.

To give you an example, on Tuesday evenings we host an open, healthy food-preparation evening in our home for our community, and we make 150-200 new recipes each year. Think about this for a minute. There are literally tens of thousands of different types of fruits and vegetables, so many that you could eat several a day each day for your entire life and never repeat any of them. There are twenty-six letters in the English alphabet, right? How many words can we make with that? Let's just say—a lot. Now jump back to the tens of thousands of different types of produce and match that with a bunch more herbs, spices, and such, and tell me just how many combinations we can come up with? Spend the balance of your life on it and you will not even begin to tap into the variety that is available.

I often say I have eaten many more foods I don't like since the change in diet than I did before, not because of lack of variety but because of the massive increase in variety! Below is a graphic showing how limited the typical western diet flavor spectrum is. I've opened up the flavor spectrum from the limiting percentage

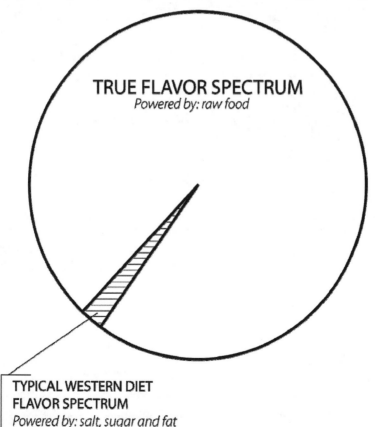

TRUE FLAVOR SPECTRUM
Powered by: raw food

TYPICAL WESTERN DIET
FLAVOR SPECTRUM
Powered by: salt, sugar and fat

our culture accepts to the limitless variety as intended by our creative and wonderful Creator God. There are some wild flavors out there! One of my favorite fruits is found in Thailand and it is called durian. It has the foulest smell of anything you can imagine, but it tastes and feels like a wonderful custard when it is going down. Our family is divided in opinion about that fruit. Nikki and Gabe won't touch it while Jake, Farrell, and I sit in the back yard (because it stinks so badly) and plow through it. Guess what? That is just one type of food and it wasn't mixed with anything. We have the opportunity to make billions of different recipes and even more variations of those recipes. The variety is endless, so don't let that be a show-stopper for you. If you try something and you don't like it, then just say so and move on to one of the seven billion or so other options available.

Whoa. I feel better now that I've got that out of the way. I hope you are encouraged when you see the massive expanse of variety designed for our diets by our Creator. Remember that He made us and our fuel. When you consider how wonderful He made our lives, would He not also have made food to be an area of great joy as well?

CHAPTER SEVEN

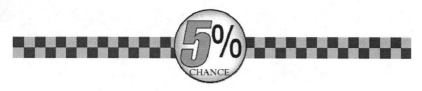

A Hallelujah Day

Of course, you will enjoy a variety of other delicious salads and cooked food dishes, but this is a basic review of what a day on The Hallelujah Diet® may look like.

Breakfast
Upon rising, take one serving of BarleyMax®, either in capsule or powder form. (Take the powder dry, dissolving it in the mouth, or mix it in a few ounces of distilled water at room temperature or with carrot/vegetable juice.) Do not have any cooked food or foods containing fiber at this meal as these hinder the cleansing process while the body eliminates accumulated toxins.

Mid-Morning
Drink an eight-ounce glass of fresh carrot/vegetable juice. If fresh juice is not available, a serving of CarrotJuiceMax™ or BeetMax™, or a piece of juicy, fresh fruit is second best.

Lunch

Before lunch, have another serving of BarleyMax®. Thirty minutes later, eat either a raw vegetable salad or raw fruit lunch. Limit your fruit consumption to 15% or less of total daily food intake. Lunch is also an all-raw meal, because cooked food is typically limited to the evening meal on The Hallelujah Diet®. (If you have cooked food at lunch, make sure dinner is an all-raw meal to maintain the benefits of The Hallelujah Diet®.)

Mid-Afternoon

Drink an eight-ounce glass of fresh carrot/vegetable juice. If fresh juice is not available, a serving of CarrotJuiceMax™ or BeetMax™, or some carrot or celery sticks are second best.

Supper/Dinner

Before supper, have another serving of BarleyMax®. Thirty minutes later, eat a large green salad comprised of leaf lettuce along with a variety of vegetables. Do not use head lettuce as it has very little nutritional value. After the salad comes the only cooked food of the day—the 15% cooked food portion that is allowed on The Hallelujah Diet®. This can be a baked potato, brown rice, legumes, steamed veggies, whole grain pasta, a veggie sandwich on whole grain bread, baked sweet potato, squash, or any other type of whole grain or vegetable. (If desired, Lunch and Supper can be switched, but only one meal should contain cooked food on any given day.)

Evening

If desired, a piece of juicy, fresh fruit or a glass of freshly extracted apple or pear juice may be consumed.

It will be much easier for you to adopt The Hallelujah Diet® once you see that the 85% raw and 15% cooked foods actually consist of an amazing array of delicious and healthy things that you may already be eating!

Response to the Hallelujah Diet® for a day from Jerrod:
As I talk through this, realize that I am at the ten year point. If you are at day one, all of this may seem incredibly foreign to you. Remember that this is a transition. You transitioned from breast

milk as a baby into the diet regime as recommended and practiced by your family. You can transition again, but give yourself some time. Don't get into a spike-and-slide routine where you make big changes and then slide back to where you were. That is a recipe for failure. Make incremental and sustainable changes you can live with, adjust to, and feel like are an advantage and not like a punishment. Always keep an eye on your next incremental change or improvement.

I don't encourage people to use capsules for the BarleyMax® unless there is some real, valid reason other than, "I don't like the flavor." It is really tough to get the same volume of nutrients from the capsules that you can from a nice, big heaping spoonful (or two as I do), because you would have to take a pile of the capsules regularly. I believe absorption into the body is quicker with the powder because it begins in your mouth. Furthermore, you get new taste buds about every three weeks if you are well hydrated, so why not just power through the taste mentally for a bit, or use something like fruit juice to reduce the fresh-cut grass flavor rather than avoiding the flavor all together? I also find that I enjoy all greens more, but that transition takes time. Realistically, I remember it taking about three months of hard-headed diligence in taking the BarleyMax® before I actually started to enjoy it.

For the kids, we began them on BarleyMax® as babies by dipping their pacifiers in the green powder and they loved it. Now they all take a spoonful of a mix of BarleyMax®, BeetMax™ and CarrotJuiceMax™ and they enjoy that, as well. For reference, I put about these amounts respectively and in this order on the spoon: ½ teaspoon, ¼ teaspoon, and 1 teaspoon.

It is uncommon for me to desire anything else early in the morning other than BarleyMax®. It can sometimes be 10am or 11am before I really begin to feel like I want something else to eat. I may have a piece of fruit, some carrot juice or a handful of nuts or maybe a combination of all of those.

FIELD NOTES: Here is what happened this morning: I generally wake between 5:00–7:00 a.m. without an alarm. I normally spend the first hour or two studying, reading and praying. Today I woke a few minutes after 6am. After laying in thought for a few minutes, I sat up, repositioned my pillow, and grabbed my ESV leather-bound Bible. I am reading through the book of Luke right now and I am fascinated by the resulting account of all the historical research done by Luke, the author of Luke and Acts—the prequel and the sequel regarding Jesus. I came out of my room at 7:30 a.m. and was greeted by Jake with a nice glass of BarleyMax® that Mommy had mixed for me. I snuggled with Gabe, who had crashed in the living room last night after we watched a race. He was just waking up. Jake joined us as well. As Gabe awoke, his first words were questions about when could we get the slot car track out and set it up (something we normally do between November and January), and where could we get some raised-bridge track pieces and a Lemans slot car to add to our already overgrown collection of cars? The conversation shifted to food soon after. I headed to my desk to get on-line and see how things were going with businesses so far that morning and I drank my BarleyMax®. After getting through the sea of initial emails for the day, I headed for the shower. When I got out, I saw the kids were having one of their favorites, chopped up honeydew and cantaloupe. They regularly waffle between who likes which. This got me thinking that I wanted a bowl of cereal, so at 9:07, I sat down to enjoy the following which took me about three minutes to whip up.

- 1 chopped peach
- ½ chopped apple
- 10 raspberries
- ¼ cup raisins
- Small handful of frozen blueberries
- ¼ cup shredded coconut, large shreds
- ¼ cup chopped walnuts
- ¼ cup puffed corn (we use puffed millet also—both sparingly, of course)
- ½-¾ cup fresh almond milk

This is a nice treat and I feel stuffed now at 9:28. I would have been fine for a couple more hours without this meal but it was an enjoyable treat.

Lunch is generally a light raw salad these days. For a long time I used to gorge on a huge salad at lunch and it was just what I needed. I wanted to feel full, and those thousands of salads my wife made were each amazing. I crave great salads every day. It is so wonderful to crave what is good for you.

We found along the way that we slept better at night if we avoided cooked foods in the evening. Ideally, we would finish our eating for the day in the early afternoon but that is still a challenge for us, mainly due to our schedules. See, even I still have my eyes on the next step. I just feel so much better on an empty stomach or a bit of a hungry feeling than always feeling topped off, full or bloated.

It is interesting to point out here that Dr. Joel Fuhrman notes in *Eat to Live* that few of us ever actually experience true hunger. I can confirm now that this is actually true. I enjoy the feeling of being slightly hungry but also enjoy eating just enough to satisfy that hunger rather than gorging or gluttony. Most of us eat out of habit, and we build an unreasonable appetite due to our poor eating habits and choices. Below is a direct quote from Dr. Fuhrman's book that I just read again and felt it was incredibly applicable here. It is speaking of people who have been living a plant-based diet for a while.

> *Even when they delay eating and get very hungry, they no longer experience stomach cramps, headaches, or fatigue accompanying their falling blood sugar. They merely get hungry and they enjoy this new sensation of hunger in the mouth and throat, which makes food taste better than ever. Many of my patients have told me that they enjoy this new sensation; they like being able to be in touch with true hunger and the pleasure of satisfying it.*

The one point I want to emphasis is that it does not require any precise measuring of calories or specific diet to maintain a thin, muscular weight. It only requires that you eat healthy food and that the hunger drive be real.

Now that you are sufficiently either freaked out by this or excited to get there, remember that it took me several years to get to this point. It is not something you should feel pressure to look for or be stressed about achieving. It is simply one of the numerous blessings set along the path for us as we align with our Creator's health basics.

As time has progressed, I was surprised to find that the less cooked food I eat, the better I feel. I still crave it and I do eat a bit of cooked food, but I always feel better on fresh, raw, organic, living, and whole food. I was talking to George a few years ago and he agreed. He felt like the diet needed to contain the 15% cooked portion more as a transitional food to get the public to accept the diet, but that it was not necessary for optimal health. I believe he spoke mainly from his own personal experiences as I am able to do now.

Interestingly, even a couple of years ago I would have disagreed if someone was to tell me that someday I would be eating 100% raw. I am not there yet but I am not completely adverse to the idea. My feeling now is that I want to eat the fuel that is going to make me feel the best, and if it is raw food then that is what I want the most of. And if someday, for a long period or short period of time, that fact lives itself out through me in an all raw diet, then I am fine with that.

I am, however, not interested in sacrificing relationships or even moments of joy with people over food. If someone were to invite our family over for dinner, and worked hard on the meal, and unknowingly included something that we didn't normally eat, I would most likely respectfully eat some of it. The exceptions to this statement would be that if it contained animal products. Then I would avoid as much of it as possible, if not all together, and if it contained excitotoxins of any kind then I would not eat it. These items are the chief offenders in my opinion, and they do cause immediate problems for many people and certainly for someone who is very clean internally like I am.

Fortunately, we nearly always have opportunities to talk about or make plans with those we socialize with. It is often a welcome teaching experience for them to try something new with us or as they prepare for us. The point here is that food is designed to bring us together in relationship as much as it is to feed and nourish our bodies. Using food to avoid being in community or using food incorrectly within relationships would be wrong in my view. Food is a by-product of life, not the point.

Socializing can really mess up eating habits. My family tends to be a lot more flexible away from home than we are at home. This is because we decided we were going to make things more simple at home in terms of choices by not stocking things in the house that are not in the four or five star range in terms of the Hallelujah Diet®. (In the book Recipes for Life, author Rhonda Malkmus has a 5-star rating system to help the reader know which recipes are healthier.) In other words, we want to be as vigilant as possible at home in our eating, snacking, and food choices. This is the core because it is the primary place we eat. Furthermore, it enables us to feel as though we are spreading our wings a bit when we travel or eat out. Clearly, eating away from home is going to be more of a challenge, and actually impossible to accurately know for sure what you are getting.

I rarely order a salad when eating out. If I do, it can be considered a huge complement because I am usually so dissatisfied with restaurant salads that I just avoid them all together. There are few places where I can get a good one. The biggest single criteria we look for when considering eating in a new place is whether they use any sort of excitotoxin (such as MSG). If so, we won't eat there. The second consideration is if they are flexible in taking their standard menu items and modifying them a bit. If we can get past these two then we are likely headed to sit down and share some time together as a family. As a side note, we would do research on-line or elsewhere prior to planning to meet someone else out. If we didn't do this, it could create an uncomfortable situation.

My advice for eating out is to take a scan over the menu to try to ascertain what they have in the kitchen. Assuming they are really flexible, you can mix and match and put together a really fun, unique meal. My favorite times are when I can just ask the waiter to request the chef "feed us" a nice vegan meal. I usually top this with a request that they avoid pasta because that seems to be a quick solution for some amateur purveyors of the kitchen. If they are comfortable with a whole food diet or a vegan diet then they can often have a lot of fun with this. If I were in their shoes, I would much rather have a restaurant where people came in, gave me an idea of what they were interested in, and how hungry they are, and then let me figure out what to create in the kitchen. Maybe someday someone will come up with a restaurant like this. Wouldn't that be fun to do as a chef?

One of the things we need to be careful of is using our schedule to avoid eating healthfully…in other words, eating out more as an excuse to binge a bit rather than going home to enjoy something more full of life. We often feel guilty for eating out, as well, because we have so much live food at home that has a definite shelf life. It is really tough for us to keep up with eating it all, so some does go to waste.

CHAPTER EIGHT

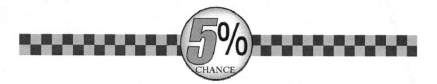

Steer Clear to Win

My hope is that this book is not characterized as a book with a bunch of "don't do's." In fact, I nearly omitted this section altogether because I feel it is much more important that you focus on what you can do rather than what you cannot or should not do. In other words, you can be very successful in just doing the right things right, for the right reasons, rather than focusing on avoiding the wrong things and giving yourself a bad attitude and overall miserable disposition.

With that said, I am going to be very brief here and give you a list of the items you should avoid and the reasons why. I also want you to see how these apply to my recipes for disease, illness, and obesity. After this list, I have highlighted the two biggest concerns I have after having lived this diet for a number of years.

The foods listed below create most of the physical problems we experience and are not a part of The Hallelujah Diet®. To have real health, eliminate them from your diet as quickly as possible.

Foods to Be Avoided

Beverages. Alcohol, coffee, tea, cocoa, carbonated beverages and soft drinks, all artificial fruit drinks including sports drinks, and all commercial juices containing preservatives, salt, and sweeteners.

Dairy. All milk, cheese, eggs, ice cream, whipped toppings, and non-dairy creamers.

Fruit. Canned and sweetened fruits, along with non-organic dried fruits.

Grains. Refined, bleached flour products, cold breakfast cereals, and white rice.

Meats. Beef, pork fish, chicken, turkey, hamburgers, hot dogs, bacon, sausage, etc.

Nuts & Seeds. All roasted and/or salted seeds and nuts. Though peanuts are not a nut but a legume, they are very difficult to digest and should also be avoided.

Oils. All lard, margarine, shortenings, and anything containing hydrogenated oils.

Seasonings. Table salt, black pepper, and any seasonings containing them.

Soups. All canned, packaged, or creamed soups containing dairy products.

Sweets. All refined white or brown sugars, sugar syrups, chocolate, candy, gum, cookies, donuts, cakes, pies, or other products containing refined sugars or artificial sweeteners.

Vegetables. All canned vegetables containing added sodium or preservatives, or vegetables fried in oil.

Once you have stopped eating the foods that will harm your health and started eating the foods that will enhance your health, you may experience some symptoms of detoxification. If you do, take heart! This means you are getting rid of toxins that have been stored in your body.

If I was told I could only name two things to avoid consuming and I had to limit my list to just these, then this is what I would say. It is tough to categorize these appropriately because I have really strong feelings about both but I don't think there is nearly as much science or personal experience around the second one as compared to the first so I will go in this order:

Animal products of any kind would be one that I would simply avoid all together. Dr. T. Colin Campbell explains, in detail, why animal products are so bad for the human body in his book, *The China Study*. It has to do with the protein and how it is processed in our bodies. It is really bad for our bodies as it leads to many of the western diseases we commonly experience as a culture. Dr. Joel Fuhrman in *Eat to Live* confirms this, and many life stories along with hundreds of scientific studies also corroborate this fact. This includes dairy, quite significantly because dairy includes the animal protein which is the chief contributor to the physical ailments. The story around fish and seafood is a bit vaguer, however. It seems the protein in these swimmers is not as big of a problem as is the toxic load from the heavy metals often found in them. I ate some fish during the first couple of years of the lifestyle change but it was infrequent and in small portions. *Eat to Live* has a chart showing which fish are more likely to contain more heavy metals.

Excitotoxins of all kinds would be next on my list. I learned everything I know about excitotoxins from Dr. Russell Blaylock in his book by the same name, that is, other than what I learned by experiencing the chemical poisoning from excitotoxins first hand on several occasions. Because I know you want to know what an excitotoxin is, I will provide a brief overview here but if you want to know details, then check out Dr. Blaylock's book.

What is an excitotoxin? An excitotoxin is an amino acid. Our bodies use a lot of amino acids regularly. The problem is that there are ways of creating amino acids in such a manner that they zoom past the protective blood-brain barrier and wreak havoc on our brain neurons (receptors). These "bad" amino acids are dubbed excitotoxins for reasons you are about to learn. The excitotoxin amino acid makes its way to the receptors in the brain that control the "feel good" signals. Interestingly enough, it is sort of like a gate. The excitotoxin holds open the gate to the receptor while calcium rushes in to cause the receptor to fire in rapid succession, sending a "feel good" signal elsewhere in the brain. Zinc and magnesium are designed to hold the gate closed in certain circumstances, but a deficiency in these minerals is common and thus leaves the receptors even more vulnerable. In other words, we are duped into thinking whatever we just did (or ate) was good for us and pleasurable. Soon after, the receptors (neurons) effected by the excitotoxin die. Here is what Dr. Blaylock says about the effects of the excitotoxins:

> *"When neurons are exposed to these substances, they become very excited and fire their impulses very rapidly until they reach a state of extreme exhaustion. Several hours later these neurons suddenly die, as if the cells were excited to death. As a result, neuroscientists have dubbed this class of chemicals 'excitotoxins.'"*

Clearly excitotoxins are something we should avoid, but where are they found? Some of the common names would be MSG, which is an acronym for monosodium glutamate or hydrolyzed protein. The problem is that many people know about the negative effects of MSG, so food manufacturers have resorted to creating new, similar substances and conveniently renaming them something else. Here is a list for your reference:

The following always contain an excitotoxin:

Autolyzed Plant Protein
Autolyzed yeast
Calcium caseinate
Gelatin
Glutamate
Glutamic acid
Hydrolyzed Plant Protein (HPP)
Hydrolyzed Vegetable Protein (HVP)
Monopotassium glutamate
Monosodium glutamate
MSG
Senomyx (wheat extract labeled as artificial flavor)
Sodium caseinate
Textured protein
Vegetable protein extract
Yeast extract
Yeast food or nutrient

The following commonly contain an excitotoxin:

Algae, phytoplankton, sea vegetable, wheat or barley grass powders

Amino acids (as in Bragg's liquid amino acids and chelated to vitamins)

Annatto

Barley malt

Bouillon

Broth

Caramel flavoring (coloring)

Carrageenan

Citric acid (when processed from corn)

Corn syrup and corn syrup solids, high fructose corn syrup Cornstarch fructose (made from corn)

Dough conditioners

Dry milk solids

Enzyme modified proteins

Fermented proteins

Flowing Agents

Gluten and gluten flour

Gums (guar and vegetable)

Lecithin

Lipolyzed butter fat

"Low" or "No Fat" items

Malt Extract or Flavoring

Malted barley (flavor)

Maltodextrin, dextrose, dextrates

Milk powder

Modified food starch

Natural chicken, beef, or pork flavoring "seasonings"

(Most assume this means salt, pepper, or spices and herbs, which sometimes it does.)

Natural flavors, flavors, flavoring

Pectin

Protease

Protease enzymes

Protein fortified milk

Protein powders: whey, soy, oat, rice (as in protein bars shakes and body building drinks)

Reaction flavors

Rice syrup or brown rice syrup

Soy sauce or extract

Soy protein

Soy protein isolate or concentrate

Spice

Stock

Ultra-pasteurized dairy products

Wheat, rice, corn, or oat protein

Whey protein isolate or concentrate

Whey protein or whey

Yeast nutrients

Anything enriched or vitamin enriched

Anything protein fortified

If that list isn't scary enough, Dr. Blaylock indicates that some excitotoxins such as aspartate and L-cysteine can be added to foods and, according to FDA rules, require no labeling at all. If you are a smoker, you should also know that some cigarettes now contain excitotoxins, and it is conceivable they could pass through the absorptive surfaces of lung tissue and enter the blood stream. There's a little more motivation to eat a plant.

This is basically the self-administered regime that I have applied to my life with great success. Of course, through the years, I have grown in my understanding and have expanded the list of things I avoid mainly out of choice rather than feeling like it was something I had to do. When I made progress in my health, I didn't feel as good when I ate certain things. Pasta is a good example. I can't remember when I last had more than a bite of pasta, but I know after I did I felt like I had a bomb in my gut. It was bad and I simply decided pasta was no longer for me in any significant quantity. Another example I like to share is my story about dropping the super-sized French fry habit. After I began the diet change, I chose to continue an infrequent McDonald's French fry habit. This continued about once or twice per quarter for a couple of years. The last time was the day I sat in the parking lot, chowing down on the fresh hot fries, and then I realized that I didn't really enjoy the flavor all that much. In fact, my mouth was a bit sticky afterwards and I can't say I felt great after eating them. For me, that was all it took. I wasn't strict about it along the way nor did I beat myself up for doing this. After all, they are vegan! The point here is that in due time you will achieve the goals you set out for, but it will take some time and diligence.

It is also important to remember my encouragement to think about what you can do rather than going too far down this path of all that you are bound from. There are more options than any of us combined will ever be able to explore and experience. Find the freedom in your lifestyle instead of focusing on the "don't do's."

CHAPTER NINE

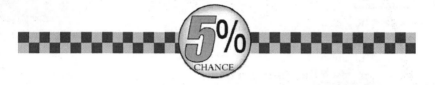

Supplements and Complements

You can optimize the effectiveness and receive maximum benefits from The Hallelujah Diet® when you combine the Hallelujah foods with these excellent supplementary products. Each day you will get vital nutrients which will help protect your immune system, as well as giving you many other health benefits.

BarleyMax®:

BarleyMax® is a blend of two of nature's most nutritionally dense foods—raw organic barley and alfalfa grass juices—in a convenient powder form.

According to Rev. George Malkmus, Lit.D., founder of Hallelujah Acres®:

"I always consume at least three teaspoons daily. One teaspoon per day may be a good starting point, and then building up to two to three teaspoons, to prevent too rapid of a cleansing reaction. If I had a serious physical problem today, I would increase my intake of BarleyMax® powder to four or more teaspoons along with six to eight 8-ounce glasses of carrot/vegetable juice daily."

The reason why Rev. Malkmus and others on The Hallelujah Diet® supplement their diets with BarleyMax® is because, for the most part, food produced today is grown in soil that lacks the nutrients the body needs for building new, strong, healthy, vital, and vibrant cells. BarleyMax® contains the juices of both raw organic barley and alfalfa, which are grown in soil that is high in minerals. This single supplement contains the widest spectrum of nutrients and the highest macro and trace mineral content possible. Dr. Michael Donaldson of the Hallelujah Acres® Foundation has performed extensive research and testing to ensure that the levels of vitamins, minerals, enzymes, and antioxidants in BarleyMax® are among the highest in the industry.

Carrot/Vegetable Juice

Freshly extracted carrot/vegetable juice made from large California juicing carrots and leafy green vegetables is extremely important in meeting daily nutritional needs. Carrots are the richest source of beta-carotene, the precursor of vitamin A, which the body can easily absorb, plus it provides a wealth of other nutritional benefits. The carrot/vegetable juice and BarleyMax® make a dynamic duo in providing the body with high-octane body fuel. As a maintenance program, consume at least two 8 ounce glasses of carrot/vegetable juice along with two to three servings of BarleyMax® daily.

If you do not have a juicer to make your own fresh carrot/vegetable juice, you can use convenient juice powders like CarrotJuiceMax™ and BeetMax, which are made from organic carrots and organic beets, contain no artificial ingredients, are naturally sweet, and provide practically all of the nutrients and live enzymes of the fresh raw carrots and beets. This makes them the perfect substitutes when fresh carrot/vegetable juices are not available.

Fiber Cleanse

Use Fiber Cleanse* during the first two to three months on The Hallelujah Diet®, taking the recommended serving before leaving for work or sometime in the late morning. The twenty-eight selected herbs and fibers are in a psyllium and flax seed base, and help cleanse the colon, restore normal bowel activity, ensure timely and efficient elimination of toxins from the body, and more— a must for achieving optimal health.

After three months, we recommend you transition to either freshly ground organic flax seed or our new B-Flax-D™ product for long-term use.

*Not recommended for pregnant or lactating women, or for long-term use.

Vitamin B12

Those following The Hallelujah Diet® should consider taking a supplement to ensure an adequate level of Vitamin B12 in the body, as this nutrient is not readily found in a primarily vegan diet. Adequate levels of B12 help the body to do the following: prevent anemia, regulate red blood cell formation, form healthy cells, metabolize fats and carbohydrates, utilize iron, prevent nerve damage, and perform many other functions properly.

The vitamins B6 and Folic Acid provide related health benefits, such as metabolizing protein, forming hemoglobin, and decreasing neural tube defects. We combined B12 with B6 and Folic Acid into a vegetarian sublingual tablet to help you get the best 1-2-3 nutritional health punch this combination can deliver. For those who are pregnant, this combination is a must for your health and that of your child.

Udo's Choice Perfected Oil Blend™

One tablespoon per day of Udo's oil, a cold-pressed blend of organic flax, sunflower, and sesame seed oils, combined with oils from oat germ and rye germ, will give you the essential omega-3 and omega-6 fatty acids the body needs to achieve and maintain good health. However, this oil should not be used for cooking. An alternative to using the Udo's oil is to take a serving of B-Flax-D™ as directed, to meet the daily needs of essential fats, vitamin D, and fiber.

Attention Men: Current research indicates that men dealing with prostate cancer may be better served by using freshly ground flax seed to meet their essential fats needs rather than the Udo's oil or flax seed oil.

Sunshine

Each sunny day, get some sunshine (approximately fifteen minutes) on as much of the skin as possible. The sun is so important in the production of vitamin D, which is critical for strong bones and muscles, a healthy immune system, and more. On days when you cannot get an adequate amount of sunshine, take the recommended serving of B-Flax-D™.

Exercise

Exercising every day for a minimum of thirty minutes is extremely important—it helps you stay physically fit and releases toxins from the body. Doing a combination of aerobic, resistance, and stretching exercises will help maximize your body's cardiovascular condition, strength, and flexibility. When first beginning an exercise regimen, doing a stretching and fast walking program is a good place to start.

When you combine these things with all the great foods of The Hallelujah Diet®, you will feel the incredible difference!

I consider BarleyMax® to be mandatory for those consuming the typical western diet or even The Hallelujah Diet® in the western culture. There are a number of reasons, but generally because it is the most nutrient-dense and most wonderful food on the planet. We cannot get perfect food even if we are eating all organic whole foods.

According to Dr. Olin Idol, though we may be able to equal or even exceed the juice quality for the BeetMax or CarrotJuiceMax™ if we get superb fresh beets and carrots, it would be nearly impossible for us to do this with BarleyMax®. The beet and carrot juices contain some organic brown rice solids which prevent the absorption of moisture and caking of the powder. BarleyMax® does not contain these added ingredients.

If we could grow our own barley grass under comparable conditions as the barley grass used for BarleyMax®, it would also be superior to our supplement. However, that simply isn't possible for most people. For those who can do it, they would be limited to a short harvest period. But we can purchase carrots and beets year round.

People may use the powders if fresh juicing isn't an option. I used primarily fresh juices but I also used powder when juicing wasn't possible. When I did, I used 2/3 carrot and 1/3 greens.

BarleyMax® is:

- Grown organically in mineral rich, heavily composted soils, watered with mineral-rich water from deep below the earth's surface.

- Barley grass and alfalfa seeds used in BarleyMax® are planted in the fall, allowing the seed to germinate and develop a significant root system throughout the late fall and winter. In early spring, the grass begins to sprout and grow very slowly in the cool temperatures, allowing for the absorption of a vast array of nutrients from the organically enriched soils. This slow growth in the cool temperatures allow for the development of a very complex sugar molecule, providing a nutrient-rich grass. The only juice powder I would recommend over fresh juice is BarleyMax®, because of this rapid growth of the wheat grass sprouts with the simple sugar and low nutrient makeup.

- The barley grass is harvested at the peak of nutrition, prior to the jointing stage that would produce the grain. Thus, the grass is free of the grain and contains no gluten (found in the grain). The mature alfalfa is utilized as the younger alfalfa sprouts contain a non-protein amino acid L-Canavanine that may be toxic in large amounts. The level of this amino acid drops dramatically as the grass matures and is not a concern in the mature grass.

- The grasses are cut, bailed, and transported immediately to the processing facility so they are not exposed to any heat. It is washed (not sanitized) and juiced. The juice is dried in a low temperature environment so the enzymes and heat-sensitive nutrients are not destroyed.

- There is virtually no fiber in BarleyMax®. It is a 100% pure juice powder with no added items such as fillers and stabilizers.

- One of the benefits of cereal grasses is something not yet fully identified called the "grass juice factor," which is attributed for supplying yet-unidentified nutritional elements that account for much of the benefit to the consumer.

- Grasses can support optimal growth and development of large mammals such as horses and cows for a full lifetime when the animals are allowed to graze on them naturally, apart from man's interference. Not only are these grasses are a complete food for these animals, they're also a good food for humans as well.

- BarleyMax® may be taken dry or with water or juices. Since it is a 100% juice powder, the nutrients have been released from the cellular structures of the grasses and are readily available for absorption regardless of the way they are consumed.

- BarleyMax® is an alkaline-forming juice.

- Many other green juice powders contain whole grass fiber which cannot be digested by man's digestive system, thus leaving the nutrients locked in the fibers. Most juice powders are processed in a way that results in most of the enzymes and heat-sensitive nutrients being destroyed.

- Growing and processing are the key factors that make BarleyMax® superior to other concentrated green products.

If you refer to Dr. Joel Fuhrman's book, *Eat to Live*, you will see a nutrient density chart on pages 120-121. The chart shows low-density foods such as refined sweets, refined oils, refined grains, cheese, and dairy at less then five points of a possible 100. Notice that nothing on the nutrient density chart scoring above fifty is any color other than green. I think this is a great indication from a scientific stand point that the more we emphasize green foods in our diet, the more healthy our bodies will be.

CHAPTER TEN

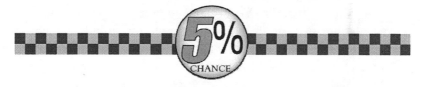

Hallelujah Acres Mission

Hallelujah Acres exists to share the health message as designed and prescribed by our Creator God to the believers in God.

There is a back story behind the mission that, to my knowledge, only a few people know. It has to do with the creation of the Hallelujah Acres privately branded products. I am one of only a handful that knows most of this story, though I don't know all the greasy details. However, I do know enough to share here and feel comfortable about it. I also know that the leadership at Hallelujah Acres have avoided sharing publicly about this because there simply was no way for them to communicate the truth accurately without making other people or companies look bad for their choices. Thankfully, I am not paid by them or any other organization but rather by you for buying this book, so consider this the "tell all" chapter...

Why would I share this? My chief goal is to get you to a point, as I am, that you can fully trust Hallelujah Acres, their teaching, their leadership, and the results from projects the Hallelujah Acres Research Foundation completes. We do not have time to know everything. We need a cornerstone of information to rely on and just be able to go to a list of FAQs to get what we need without having to know all the backdrop information. Hallelujah Acres quite literally exists for this reason.

The problem is that as a culture, we are not willing to pay rightly for this information. We are willing to buy some books and videos but books are low margin (limited profit), and informational videos and the like are expected more and more to be streamed and either free or nearly free. So, Hallelujah Acres generates a good portion of their budget from the sale of products and equipment. With that statement I want to be very clear that Hallelujah Acres has not, did not, and hopefully will not ever create products for the sole purpose of generating revenue. They only produce, brand and supply items that are necessary and helpful to each of us that is attempting to follow a healthy, biblically-based diet regime such as the Hallelujah Diet®.

Ok, I feel like I just wrote a legal disclaimer so now I will get on with the story!

A few years ago Hallelujah Acres began producing and selling their own privately labeled products. In business, this is done for a number of reasons. If you ever shop at Trader Joe's, you will see that most of the products on their shelves are privately labeled with their name. This does not mean Trader Joe's actually has a manufacturing plant that produces all these products. What it means is that they agree with other makers that they will package their existing products or new products they agree to make in special privately labeled packaging. This gives uniqueness to the product in the marketplace and eliminates the general public from comparing apples to apples in things like price and quality. It also allows Trader Joe's to switch vendors without their customers knowing. If you shop at Costco, you know that this is one of the things that is super annoying because they begin carrying something that you really like and then before you know it, that item is gone altogether or replaced by something that is, at least in the purveyor's eyes, of lesser quality than the previous product. So, what does all of this have to do with Hallelujah Acres?

Hallelujah Acres leadership and staff rightfully uphold the responsibility of providing the very best information, supplies, and equipment known or available to their consumers (you and I) as the most important activity in their ministry. Note that this does not circumvent the purpose of life and ministry which is to be on the mission for and with Jesus Christ. Hallelujah Acres takes their responsibility very seriously. They truly want the best for you and me. I have spent time and have relationships with the leadership at Hallelujah Acres. They are genuine lovers of Christ, great leaders of integrity, and wonderful brothers and sisters who have devoted their lives to ensuring you and I have the information we need to achieve the highest level of success possible in our physical and spiritual lives.

So, why did Hallelujah Acres begin privately labeling their own products? Where did this all start? For many years, Hallelujah Acres recommended we purchase another green powder product sold through a multi-level marketing organization. The income from this relationship was necessary for Hallelujah Acres to balance their budget on a monthly basis. This income represented the majority of the income that Hallelujah Acres earned. It was a very big deal.

Not long after the turn of the last century, Dr. Michael Donaldson of the Hallelujah Acres Foundation completed some research analyzing many green powder products. Around this same time, the multi-level company they were working with announced privately they had completed a new formula that they were planning to begin offering under a new name. Upon review of this formula and samples, it was found that this product was greatly inferior to what Dr. Donaldson had found in what would become BarleyMax®.

Of course the leadership of Hallelujah Acres presented their findings to the multi-level marketing company. To their surprise, the option to use this superior product was rejected due to business circumstances related to profitability around their new product as compared to what would become BarleyMax®. In other words, they stood to make more money on their own formula. What this shows is that their priority was profit first and at best, product quality was second, but could have been third or worse. You will find the same is true for most food producers.

Deflated and shocked, the Hallelujah Acres leadership returned with some tough decisions to prayerfully make. However, these decisions were swift and decisive. They quickly came to an agreement with the producer of what is now BarleyMax® and began working and planning to privately label all of the products offered by Hallelujah Acres. This would give them full rein to always ensure the very best formulas were used and offered to those who know and trust Hallelujah Acres for products and information.

The transition was a tumultuous time because of the reaction by the multi-level marketing company, and some of the people that chose not to trust and continue to follow Hallelujah Acres leadership. The income stream from the sale of the legacy green powder product was terminated immediately by the multi-level marketing company, which left Hallelujah Acres in a difficult and uncomfortable situation. Thankfully they trusted God and pressed forward with what they knew would be best in the long term for you, me, and the mission of the organization. I don't know what the personal investment was on the part of Hallelujah Acres or the leadership, but I can guess that everything would have been put at stake if that is what it took to make this transition.

The result was that many of the people who were previously recommending the green powder sold through this multi-level organization did in fact switch to BarleyMax®. Like Hallelujah Acres, they were more interested in ensuring the people received the very best quality product available rather than personal financial gain. Hallelujah Acres did implement a payment plan, albeit not a multi-level marketing program, to ensure that anyone recommending the use of Hallelujah Acres products received appropriate compensation. It is important that this continues.

There are thousands of people throughout the world who desire to invest their lives in sharing this good news through their communities. In order to do this, they need an avenue for income to support their families' needs.

Unfortunately, not everyone made the switch. This made for a very tough transition and somewhat divided many of the people following Hallelujah Acres. The multi-level marketing company, along with their faithful marketers, literally made up stories and began openly bashing Hallelujah Acres. This was hurtful and discouraging to the Hallelujah Acres leadership, but they stayed the course and made a conscious decision to not respond to the complaints by the opposition because they felt as if they would be stooping to their level and adding fuel to the fire.

Years have passed since then, and I am happy to say that Hallelujah Acres has continued to research and bring innovating improvements to BarleyMax®. They have also added an entire line of whole foods and supplemental products to support people at their various stages of growth and healing. I think it is important to understand that BarleyMax® has been remixed and improved more than once since this time. What this proves is that Hallelujah Acres really isn't in this for money first, but to truly improve and provide the very best products available even if it comes at direct expense to them. During all of these improvements, the cost of BarleyMax® has remained steady, thus the research and development costs were borne by the manufacturer, grower, and Hallelujah Acres.

You can be sure when you purchase something with the Hallelujah Acres seal on it that it has been tested and proven to be the very best possible product available or known at the current time. You can also count on them to continue to innovate and improve the products they already have. Rather than rest on the research of yesterday, they continue to invest and improve on our behalf. To this I say, hallelujah!

So, hopefully now you can understand why I am so comfortable trusting the research and suggestions that come from Hallelujah Acres. They deserve our support in the purchase of products and equipment. The greatest value we gain from the organization is education and knowledge for which we don't actually pay.

They will openly admit they do not know everything. Saying so would be arrogance, given the circumstances of our world. We live in a broken, fallen world that is toxic in nature, and recommendations for optimal health are moving targets at best. I enjoy the transparency Hallelujah Acres demonstrates. For example, a couple years ago they completed some research regarding excess use of distilled water. They realized scientifically and in practice that it would be best to add some liquid minerals back into the distilled water. The reason for this is that the distilled water has the ability to strip minerals from our bodies because it is devoid of them when it enters our body directly out of the distiller. It is great to distill the water, but best to add the liquid minerals back into the distilled water before consumption. Hallelujah Acres openly admitted that their previous recommendation for years to use distilled water was flawed, therefore it was better to add the minerals after distilling.

A year or two later, they completed additional research on the water ionizing machines that basically adjust the pH level of water. The thinking with these machines is that by increasing the pH level they can decrease the toxicity or acid environment within the body. This is actually true, but the big problem is that the ionizing machines do not remove all of the toxins that the distillation process does. Thus, the very best methods possible now would be to distill tap water, then run that water through a water ionizing machine, and then, before consuming, add the liquid minerals. The struggle with this is that there is no equipment readily available that would enable anyone in a typical residential situation to be able to distill and then ionize the same water. If someone could build this sort of method right now, it would be the best known processed water we could consume.

Before I get back to the point of this water discussion, I want to mention that the very best water filter and mineralizer is a plant. That's right—the best source of water is through fresh, raw, organic, whole plants. I struggled with dehydration in the early years of my primarily plant-based diet because I didn't generally drink plain water. At that time, I was only eating maybe a little over 50% raw, and I was not getting enough water of any kind.

In this example of water, Hallelujah Acres did a great job on our behalf of being fully transparent and willing to admit tangibly that they, like us, still have a lot to learn. The more research they are able to do on our behalf, the better it will be for each of us who count on them for direction, instruction, and guidance. Similar to the circumstances around green powder products, Hallelujah Acres will do what is good for the people that count on them with their lives, regardless of the impact to their bank account. That is not something many organizations can say is true or real today.

CHAPTER ELEVEN

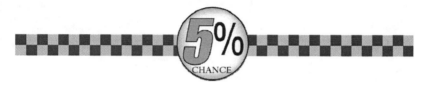

Living In Community

I am frequently asked about the process I used to achieve optimal health, specifically how I beat cancer and what that looked like on a daily basis. I hope this handbook gives you a good scope of what my days look like. However, here I want to focus in on the piece related to living in community.

There are generally two areas of concern that I see. First, I see that people are growing in a culture that is bent on separation rather than unity If you question this, then show me one piece of technology or revolutionary improvement of the last century that brings us together and I will show you a hundred that draw us apart.

Secondly, I see that we tend to use community as a crutch for living in unhealthy ways. This is not limited to diet by any means, but we certainly tend to be gluttonous when we meet. The heart behind serving each other sumptuous food is wonderful, but would not the result be even better if we took the time to think more holistically in regard to not just how the food will taste for our guests, but also on the resulting impact to the body? We tend to set negative examples rather than positive ones for each other. We need to challenge each other to live for the right reasons. Again, food is just one piece of a bigger equation here

Hebrews 10 is clear that we should not give up meeting together. Life happens when we meet together. The Bible, as a whole, should be translated in terms of community. It was not written (for the most part) to individuals, but it was written to groups of people. It should be contextualized in a similar way.

When we do meet together, we share our gifts, our experiences, and our talents. When we stay alone or segregate ourselves, we tend to keep the lights low and huddle around making excuses for why we are not doing the things we should be doing. My challenge here is for you to get with a community of people you can grow with. If you don't see a community you can join, then lead!

Years ago, we realized we needed a community, so we began hosting weekly classes in our church. After a year, we got fed up with the low attendance and stopped. It was just too much work and we didn't see any practical point of continuing. We were not building community and therefore the community was not growing. After a few weeks, my mom came to us and asked if we would start it up again but in our home. It was a great idea— much easier. And guess what? People showed up! Now we have a packed house nearly every Tuesday evening throughout the year. We ask for a five dollar donation for those that can afford it, and we usually try 150-200 new recipes a year—some we like and others we don't. When we are traveling, others will host in our home in our absence (it is usually my mom but there are other regulars as well). It is a wonderful community and we have had literally hundreds of people roll through those evenings over the years.

The point with all this is that you simply will not be successful with this if you are attempting to be like an island instead of a community. We are designed to fellowship (to share life together). Remember that life happens when we are together!

One final point I want to make about community and the Tuesday night food prep is that, although we get fifteen to forty-five people on any given Tuesday evening, we would do it if it was just my family. Seriously, it is really enjoyable for just a few of us to come together or even just our family. The kids love the kitchen, and it is a wonderful time to try new recipes and enjoy some time together catching up and working out our lives together. It is also a very comfortable, non-threatening setting for people to visit and peek into real Christian lives. Our food does not make us Christian but it does serve as a wonderful introduction. It is not uncommon that we find ourselves helping people physically, and that in turn leads to the more important work of helping them grow spiritually.

Church Community Is Typically Unhealthy
The church is completely devoid of emphasis on one of the most pernicious sins that ails our body and the culture in which we live. To fully grasp this it will be helpful to know that the dirty word "sin" is quite simply allowing one of our false idols to dethrone God in our lives. I don't believe our lifestyle choices are the chief sin or folly of the body of Christ. It is just one of the many ways in which we dethrone God from His rightful position. Nevertheless, we hear teaching that references food and gluttony, yet never takes it a step further. When the preaching and corporate worship is complete, what do we do? Head to the lobby for donuts and coffee or out to enjoy a meal together. All of this is wonderful and these are designed activities by God, but is it necessary to feed the ills of the flesh (the very things that cause disease) in order to enable key relationships in our lives to flourish, or for us to find pleasure in life? Couldn't we be doing the very same actions with the substitution of more healthy options?

Living Cross-Culturally
Whenever you do something counter-culture, you are more than likely right!

You may be surprised to hear that Nikki and I received only two home dinner invitations during the ten year period after I was diagnosed. Was this because we had recently gotten married, started having kids, diagnosed with cancer, or because we ate some funky diet that no one really understood? The answer seemed obvious. It was partly because all the changes in our lives seriously impacted the friendships we had. However, most of it was due to the fact we just didn't eat along the lines of our culture. We believe people chose to avoid that for two reasons. First, it was because they didn't want a spotlight illuminating their diet choices, and secondly, because they just didn't know what food to make or how to prepare it.

This could have been discouraging for us but we were so busy having people over to our place that we really didn't even notice it until several years had passed. We then made a conscious choice to begin attempting to reach out even more to build some more of these vital relationships. We found that once people got to know us and understood why we live the way we do, they became very interested in learning more about it. Sound familiar? This lines up perfectly with how we are to show people the love of God, right?

Living cross-culturally is fun. Being normal is boring! Most of my life when I was growing up, people called me weird (what was up with that?). I would go home upset, and my mom confirmed it by telling me that "I was not weird—I was just different." Being different somehow made me feel better at the time. As I look back, though, my mom was right on the mark. She taught me a great lesson by confirming I was actually different and that was okay. We are all different. We are all uniquely made. We all have a special combination of attributes that make us, well…us. Isn't it nice to know, however, that we have a loving God who supports, encourages, and loves each of us in the very same way? And, that same Creator made a path for each of us that is perfect, and it's the same in terms of physical health and healing. Find it. Live it. Enjoy it!

CHAPTER TWELVE

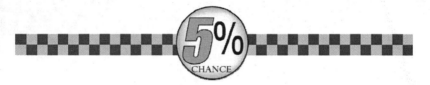

Lighten Up!

Contrary to what you may think, this chapter isn't actually about weight loss. In fact, you won't find a chapter in the book that specifically addresses weight loss. The omission of it is purposeful on my part. As a culture we are too focused on the wrong things, and we are generally unwilling to ask the right questions and face what may at times be the painful truth. Furthermore, we are not the least bit interested in enlightenment. Education, I mean. If I had titled this chapter "Education," you might have skipped it because that is the way our culture is programmed.

About fifty years ago, when C.S. Lewis wrote *The Screwtape Letters*, he, in my estimation, accurately predicted one of the problems with a democratic society. As I dive into this, know that I am the strongest proponent for a republic society, the type of system we have here in the United States. Of the choices available, or that have so far been attempted, a republic seems to yield the overall best advantages and results. What I am attempting to demonstrate is that mankind has always had, and will continue to have, a built-in propensity to avoid what we need—education.

In section two, Mr. Lewis writes: For *"democracy" or the "democratic spirit" (diabolical sense) leads to a nation without great men, a nation mainly of sub-literates, full of the cocksureness which flattery breeds on ignorance, and quick to snarl or whimper at the first hint of criticism. And that is what Hell wishes every democratic people to be. For when such a nation meets in conflict a nation where children have been made to work at school, where talent is placed in high posts, and where ignorant mass are allowed no say at all in public affairs, only one result is possible.*

C.S. Lewis had the same concern I have, and one I believe we are seeing played out in the western culture right in front of our eyes. We are more concerned about our comfort than we are about our fundamental future. We think more about what's going on today than we do about preparing a better place for tomorrow.

Our short-sightedness plays out in our lack of desire for education. As a culture, we are trained to "do school" when we are little. Education beyond K-12 is generally optional in nature. We largely attend college to get a degree in some career field, but beyond that, there's really no concern for continuous on-going education."

The chief issue is that it seems we value our comfort and our vices over our responsibility to lead from the current for the sake of the future. If we had a healthy respect for the responsibility that is, at least currently, on our shoulders then we would have less apathy and entitlement and more action, indignation, and entrepreneurship.

The forefathers of this great country of America knew full well they could not stop the process of education in their own lives. The thought was not even conceivable. I would suggest that the position of most citizens of our time would have quite literally made them ill. As a veteran, I often wonder if the ultimate price that so many soldiers paid was at least partly in vain. Below is a quote from John Adams, our nation's second president and father of the sixth president.

Laws for the liberal education of youth, especially for the lower classes of people, are so extremely wise and useful that to a humane and generous mind, no expense for this purpose would be thought extravagant.

I must study politics and war that my sons may have liberty to study mathematics and philosophy. My sons ought to study mathematics and philosophy, geography, natural history, naval architecture, navigation, commerce, and agriculture in order to give their children a right to study painting, poetry, music, architecture, statuary, tapestry, and porcelain.

There are two types of education. One should teach us how to make a living, and the other how to live.

John Adams understood the need for education quite clearly. As I did a bit more researching, I found many quotes from notable people, including our founding fathers. It's exciting for me to share these quotes with you. These people, so much more distinguished than I, make my points more eloquently than I ever could.

If a nation expects to be ignorant and free, in a state of civilization, it expects what never was and never will be. – Thomas Jefferson

Education's purpose is to replace an empty mind with an open one. – Malcolm Forbes

We are shut up in schools and college recitation rooms for ten or fifteen years, and come out at last with a bellyful of words and do not know a thing. – Ralph Waldo Emerson

The recipe for perpetual ignorance is: be satisfied with your opinions and content with your knowledge. – Elbert Hubbard

Life is not divided into semesters. You don't get summers off and very few employers are interested in helping you find yourself. – Bill Gates

People will pay more to be entertained than educated. – Johnny Carson

The highest form of ignorance is when you reject something you don't know anything about. – Wayne Dyer

Hopefully you will see that I want to motivate you to think about life as a process of learning. These men did not make these statements from the paradigm of an eighteen- or twenty-two-year education. They clearly recognized that education begins with each new day. Day by day, the lessons of life are actually the sessions of our continuing education. You are never too old to take a class on-line or at the local college. You are welcome to visit local businesses to learn from them, or volunteer to fill a need in your community. If you are interested in history, then sitting with, and listening to, (even filming!) the elderly, is critical to the documentation of what has happened prior to our birth.

In order for you to be successful in making the right changes that will lead to health and vitality for you, your family and the future generations of your family, each of us must commit to continuing to allow education to be a vital part of our days. What that looks like for you may be different than for me, but the end result is the same.

Equally important is the blessing of revelation. Revelations are pure and utter gifts from God. The effect of revelation is no different than true education. The only difference is that we don't have to work for revelation. When you look at the history of our country, and likely many of the people who have surrounded your life, you will no doubt see many people who relied on God for inspiration through revelation. Samuel Adams, George Walton, Benjamin Franklin, and John Hancock, along with all of the founding fathers of this country, kneeled together in prayer on the congressional floors of this great country. Their prayers are documented in the historical records. They understood the value of revelation, and they respected the God who so generously provides it in a way that is difficult for us to fully grasp.

Our lives begin to end when we lose interest in furthering our vision through education and revelation.

Weight Loss & Calories

Since you probably thought that, because of the name, this chapter was going to be about weight loss or weight issues, I will give you just a brief bit of information about that.

First of all, we need to gain a proper understanding of this entire topic. We should attempt to be content with our physical body as it is, yet maintain stoic focus on where we are going and where we want to be. What I mean is, do not condemn yourself for your present state. You can't change the choices you made in the past, but you can change what you do today and all the days that still lie ahead. Self-condemnation is unhealthy and can be used to simply create an excuse to slip back into unhealthy patterns.

Secondly, we need to gather a proper understanding of what weight we should be. I believe this varies from one person to the next, but in general, it is safe to say we can use a range. I like the tool that Dr. Joel Fuhrman shared in *Eat to Live*:

> **Women:** *Approximately ninety-five pounds for the first five feet of height and then four pounds for every inch thereafter. Example: A 5'6" female should weigh approximately 119 pounds.*
>
> 5'4"   95 + 16 = 111
>
> 5'6"   95 + 24 = 119
>
> **Men:** *Approximately 105 pounds for the first five feet of height and then five pounds for every inch thereafter. Example: A 5'10" male should weight approximately 155 pounds.*
>
> 5'9"   105 + 45 = 150
>
> 6'0"   105 + 60 = 165

With this information in hand, we can establish some general guidelines for where we should be with our weight; however, worrying about a number on the scale isn't the point. As I reiterate further on, this and calorie counting is a waste of time. Let's put our focus on the right things and allow the results to land where they may. When you do figure out your weight range using Dr. Fuhrman's numbers, put it in an envelope and never look at it again, because it doesn't matter. Please, if you are one of the many that do need to drop a few pounds, don't get caught in the undercurrent of living for a certain weight. You miss out on the joy today has if you are living for someday. You shouldn't target a certain weight as your goal, but rather a healthy lifestyle. When you do that, your body will naturally respond.

You can also throw calorie-counting out with the bathwater. There is no good reason to count calories if you are eating a primarily raw, whole food, or plant-based diet. Let me explain why. When you eat a bag of chips, you can manage to pound the whole bag and still be hungry because your stomach did not register any nutrition. It is sifting through what you are eating and it isn't finding anything of real value. Therefore, the signal to stop eating is simply not sent until you begin to feel the uncomfortable pressure of overeating. This is really not good but tends to be the way we eat in the west. We eat what is set before us, right? If we don't feel the pressure then we may opt for something extra or a dessert. Either way, we generally get some sort of feeling of physical fullness. To me, full is simply the absence of a reminder. My whole body will scream at me if I get too hungry. I know what true hunger feels like. Interestingly enough, one would think during times like this that I would need to eat a huge meal to overcome such a loud and annoying call for nourishment. You would be wrong. I just need a few bites and it all goes away. It will likely return quickly if I don't eat very much, but because I eat foods my body recognizes, we are able to communicate with one another freely. It tells me what it needs and I give it something recognizable. It tells me when to stop and I naturally lose interest in eating. Yes, I said, naturally and without thought, I stop eating and walk away from the food. Cool, huh?

Think about a meal as a literal walk through the garden. There would be no plates or forks, right? So, how much would you pick? Well, if you were on a dinner walk, you would hopefully have someone enjoyable with you like your spouse, some friends, or family members. You would walk, talk, and pick whatever you wanted. You would be chiefly focused on food at the beginning because you would be hungry, but then as you lost interest in your food, your focus would turn to each other. You'd continue to walk right past most of the food hanging all around you. There would be no dishes or leftovers. Also, there would be no overeating or counting calories. Wouldn't it be neat to have a garden that you could take dinner walks in, and a family that would want to do it with you? Maybe this is a new restaurant concept...

With that said, at some point in the distant future (very distant if you have a lot of weight to lose), you may get to check that envelope and when you do, it will be fun. I lost about forty pounds in the first year after I made the change in my diet and lifestyle. About four years later, I lost another twenty pounds and now I am fine-tuning my muscle tone and weight to take another few pounds off my weight. I have always wanted to see my stomach muscles so that is something I am attempting at the moment. I had a trainer tell me it wasn't possible, but I refuse to believe that. The key to success is enjoying the process, not dreading it.

Cleansing – Frequency
Many people ask, but most don't have the guts. Everyone wants to know if they poop often enough, and is the consistency correct. If there is some pain or blood, is that normal? (No, it should not be normal, if you are wondering.) Interestingly enough, nearly everything you ever need to know about your physical body can be found with close analysis of your stool. So, the thinking on this is most certainly on the right track.

Transfer time is a measurement of the period of time from the beginning point when you eat through to evacuation of the bowels. This includes travel time through the body. The body is like a donut. You could say our digestive system is in our body, but the food that travels through it is never actually inside the body. It is inside the donut hole, sure, but it doesn't actually enter the body. It is just acted upon by the digestive system. It is either hydrated or dehydrated depending upon the stage in the process. So just how long does this process take and how often should it happen?

The digestive system is the tool to provide your body with nourishment. Many people see it as an extraction tool, and it does work as that, but that isn't the primary function. What I mean is that we see it as a machine to extract the nutrition from the things that we eat. Case in point: You eat a hamburger and think that your body will pull the nutrients from the lettuce, tomato, and ketchup, and of course the ever important protein from the meat, (that part is a lie in case you don't know yet—refer back to Chapter 8 under "Animal Products"), and then send it into your blood stream and throughout your body for whatever all those various organs and internal machines need such things for... right?

Unfortunately, that is the way most of us use the digestive system. It is actually designed to quickly capture the nutrients, which are chiefly mechanically extracted with our teeth in our mouth where nutrient absorption begins. There is some minor chemical breakdown that happens in our stomach, but not nearly as much as we commonly burden our stomach with. In other words, the right foods provide nutrients that are "plug & play" with our bodies. The stomach, and the rest of the system, doesn't need to take a lot of action to extract the nutrition.

I will use myself as an example since my body has been a living laboratory for ten years. Well, actually forty years if you count all the years I was eating like the billboards tell us to.

I head to the water closet every time I eat. It is a natural reaction for you body to clean out the old and make space for the new. The actual transit time should be well below twenty-four hours. Any guess what the typical transit time is for a westerner's diet? It's about seventy-two hours, or three days. So here is something else to think about: what happens to a bunch of fresh raw produce if you put it in the blender, and then let it sit out at room temperature for twenty-four hours? Not much right? In fact, it will most definitely still contain some life. Now think about the burger. If you blend that up (you will naturally have to add some soda pop so it will blend properly in the blender, right?) and set it out on the counter at room temperature for three days, what is it going to look like or smell like?

The problem is that certain foods make your digestive system sluggish, and it does not push as aggressively as it normally would. This is caused primarily by foods low in fiber. Did you know animal products do not contain a bit of fiber? Fiber is what activates the contractions within your intestines. It keeps things moving on through. Produce is full of fiber and water-packed with essential nutrients. The nutrient-packed water is the life blood of the plant. The fiber is just the carrier, so wouldn't it make sense it would cause your intestines to contract and push it through by design?

Your intestines are designed to be a one-way tool. Once the food passes a certain point, toxins and additional water should be added to the intestines, but nothing should be coming from the other direction. Everything should be on a one-way train to the light at the end of the tunnel. If the sludge sits in your digestive system for days, then it has the opportunity to enable toxins to enter back into the body.

So, how do you increase the trips to the outhouse? Eat more fiber! It will excite your intestines, and encourage the movement of much of the muck and pus that builds up from tons of simple carbohydrates and animal protein. Talk about an easy way to drop a few pounds. Just go on a raw, plant-based diet for a few days. There are also some herbs that can help stimulate the bowels into action. Hallelujah Acres has an herbal fiber blend that works really well. If you persist in eating a western diet, then you may consider a periodic cleanse with something like this. I am not saying it is good to eat like our culture does, but the idea of all that goo building up on the inside is worse to think about.

Since our discussions have landed us in the southern regions of our bodies, some of you may know of or wonder about the cause of rectal itching. It is caused by parasites (more toxins) escaping (being forced out) during the natural detoxification process. It isn't supposed to last long, but can be expected if you make some improvements in your eating habits as your body begins to clean house. It is gross, but it should be encouraging to know they are on their way out instead of being allowed to remain.

A diet you will most certainly hear about, if you have not already, is "The Full Plate Diet." I have studied it briefly, but have no affiliation with the organization. What I can say, from what I have seen thus far, is that they are likely going to gain a strong following. In general, from what I have read, they do encourage people to move in a healthy direction. The concern I have is that they don't seem to provide much structure for people who want to go beyond some fairly basic and simple changes. They seem to think people are likely just going to make minor changes, yet continue to live and eat according to our culture. They seem to be making tangible sense of the dimmer vs. light switch I discussed earlier in the book. "The Full Plate Diet" is really based solely on that methodology, and for that reason, I believe they will succeed greatly because they make the transition from the standard American diet to "The Full Plate Diet" seem so easy. They are also taking advantage of many on-line marketing tools and massive social networking functionality for those following the diet.

CHAPTER THIRTEEN

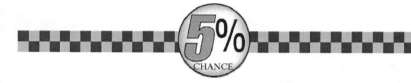

Q&A With Nikki

1) **How did you feel when I was diagnosed (re: When we received the diagnosis...)?**

   I was totally devastated. We had just been married two years, had both quit our jobs in the past six months, our insurance did not cover us in this case, and we were hoping to start our family. After the initial shock of it all, I did find peace in knowing God had a plan for our lives and that this must somehow play into that. At the time, neither Jerrod nor I had any idea of how that would be. However, God has continually and amazingly opened the doors for our story to be shared.

2) **What has been your greatest struggle with this diet and lifestyle change?**

   First a little history on how I grew up eating. It was just my mom and me. I never thought about it at the time, but she didn't like fruit or veggies. We never had any in the house, not that I would have eaten them then, even if we had. With that said, my diet consisted of hamburgers, pizza, soda, and candy bars. The only salad we ever had was something my mom would make with a big piece of iceberg lettuce laid on a plate, a banana sliced in half on top of it, with that topped with mayonnaise and walnuts. Until I met Jerrod, I had never had many different vegetables, including broccoli or asparagus. My greatest struggle with this diet and lifestyle choice is dealing with an addiction I have to soda and not giving into the cravings I have for the food that I grew up with, even though I know how bad they are and know what is good. It is also a struggle knowing that people look up to me, because I am married to Jerrod. I don't feel like I should be looked up to because I'm dealing with these other issues. It makes me feel hypocritical sometimes. I believe 100% in this program and what a difference it can make. I just feel badly I don't always live the example for people to follow.

Another challenge for me was taking the BarleyMax®. I had a hard time with that. When I was using the capsules, it wasn't difficult at all, because I couldn't taste it. However, mixing the powder with liquid and drinking it is a better way to get it into your system. I also struggled with consuming a high percentage of raw food, and eating most of that in veggies. Our family, like most in our culture, has propensity towards cooked food. A little is fine but it can easily become more than we really want it to be. We do a lot of salads, but even in our salads we use tomatoes, cucumbers, avocados, and bell peppers, which are technically all fruits (Hallelujah Acres recommends the majority of the 85% raw be vegetables vs. fruits).

Jerrod: Nikki is wonderful and I am so proud of her for what she has done in terms of diet and lifestyle choices for our family and herself. I try to remind her that she has made it 70% of the way from where she was rather than her tendency to focus on the distance she still has to travel.

Possibly not unlike you, Nikki wasn't facing a terminal illness like I was when she began this journey. I was. I often tell people that the choices on a day-to-day basis were not as difficult for me as they will be for those who choose this "because it is right." You see, every time I lifted my fork, I thought one of these two words, "life" or "death." I knew that if I chose "death" too many times, that was going to be the result for me. I am proud of Nikki and of you for making these tough but rewarding changes!

3) **Being Jerrod's wife, what challenges have you faced to try to accommodate his desires within the diet?**
Jerrod likes a variety when it comes to his food. For instance, when we make salads, sometimes he will walk into the pantry and open the spice drawer and just start pouring different spices into his salad. This is not my style. I'm not overly comfortable in the kitchen. I did not spend any time there while I was growing up, and I just don't feel like I do a good job when I am there. Needless to say, I use recipes and do not stray far from the instructions.

4) **What would you say to someone who is facing serious physical problems?**
Do it! What do you have to lose? There are so many testimonies of how this program has turned people's lives around from death's door. Our own family has examples of how we've benefited from this and the drastic changes that have taken place. As a trial before really committing to this lifestyle, our entire family (moms, brothers, and sisters) did it with us. We were seeing if it really worked. My mom, who is diabetic and has a list of other health issues, was one of the ones who tried it. In three months, she lost six dress sizes, was off her high blood pressure medicine and almost all the way off of her diabetes medicine. Unfortunately, she didn't want to make the permanent change and chose not to continue. She quickly gained all of the weight back, plus some. As she ailed from her diseases, she had to have all of the toes on her right foot and eventually most of her foot

amputated because of diabetes. I sure wish she would have stayed on the program.

5) What was the pregnancy process like without animal products?

I didn't find it difficult going without animal products during my three pregnancies. The hardest part was dealing with midwives, doctors, concerned friends, and family who didn't understand why we've made the choice not to include that in our diet. All three of our kids have been very healthy since birth and have never had any animal products.

6) What special accommodations have you adopted in order to live and raise kids in a culture that is so contrary to the lifestyle our family chooses to live?

We bring our own food with us pretty much everywhere we go. When we travel, we have a cooler full of food for us to eat. When we fly, we stop at a supermarket and go shopping to load up our hotel room. When we go out, we are very selective and make sure the places we go are accommodating to our needs. We have had great luck with Mexican, Thai, and Soup & Salad restaurants (as long as we make sure they don't use MSG). Our kids are often invited to friends' houses for parties or play dates. I make sure we bring our lunch or our own treats. For the birthday parties, we are always asked, "What do you do about the birthday cake?" Our kids love fruit leathers, snack bars, and other healthy treats they don't get at home very often. When we go to parties, I bring those along for them to have instead of cake. They have not once asked to have cake instead of their treats. At the last party we went to, a friend of Gabe's (our oldest) asked if he could have what Gabe was having instead of the cake. Lucky for him I brought extra!

7) When talking with people who are facing a difficult situation physically, what are your top three recommendations for action steps they can take now?

Stop eating meat and dairy products, start drinking carrot juice, and start taking BarleyMax®.

Jerrod: I would suggest a strong approach to self-education as well. There are many times when my willpower may have failed, but the knowledge came through to assist me in doing what was right.

8) **What do you think your life would look like if you had not learned about the Hallelujah Diet and Lifestyle®?**
From the diagnoses the doctors were giving us, I know we wouldn't have three gifts from God that we have right now (Gabe, Farrell and Jake). I also think it is very likely I would have been a widow at a young age. I am so thankful and grateful to the Hallelujah Acres organization for their support and friendship and for Jerrod's Uncle Brad and Aunt Patti for introducing us to the program.

9) **What is it like being married to a racecar driver?**
It is very exciting, but at the same time very stressful. Jerrod is a great driver, but that doesn't help the knot my stomach gets into when he gets in the car.

10) **What is your favorite food?**
I love to snack on tomatoes, cucumbers, nuts, and homemade guacamole. We also enjoy having cheeseless pizza every now and then as a special treat.

Raising Healthy Kids
Since Nikki was willing to share in this section, I thought it would also be good to talk about raising healthy kids. We have a ton to learn in this area but we have traveled with a lot of good instruction. Some has been just good basic common sense and some has been from others. One great source we have used is a book called Pregnancy, Children & the Hallelujah Diet® by Dr. Olin Idol. In it, Dr. Idol covers many of the nutritional questions we have faced.

Immunizations
Immunization is a delicate and often stress-filled subject, mostly due to all the cultural pressure to stay within the typical social lines. It seems nearly every month now we are hearing a story of an otherwise well-meaning family being torn apart because of their unwillingness to submit to conventional medical treatments.

Granted, some of these stories are a bit far out there, and clearly these people are completely ignorant and misled in terms of true nutrition. The reality is that Nikki and I are lumped into the same category by the population, and more importantly by the courts of the land. If one of our kids was to fall ill, for example, to the swine flu, and it was found out that we refused immunizations, then we could quickly find ourselves as the family of the month on national television facing jail time or worse, being forced to subject our family's bodies to deadly toxins.

Needless to say, this has been a topic of discussion and prayer within our home for many years. In many ways, we would prefer no one knew we refused immunizations. However, we also know we must lead with the truth, not from the middle. I realize some risk of backlash comes from this. I also realize that for many people, a blanket disregard for immunizations is possibly not the correct option. If, for example, a family is not going to commit to a diet such as the Hallelujah Diet® or something similar, and they plan to continue to consume foods and toxins that deflate the immune system from performing at the very highest level, then God only knows what the best solution is for them in terms of immunizations. For some, it is conceivable they may benefit from the drugs called immunizations. Others may die because of the toxic load. If you are not a parent yet, or if your kids have grown, and you were not faced with this for whatever reason, you can now begin to see why this is such a big deal to those of us who are in the middle of it.

Pregnancy

The ability to achieve a healthy pregnancy is growing tough and seems impossible for some today. We have first-hand experience with more than one couple who has had success getting pregnant once they got their diet in line to balance their systems. It is an honor to know that some children are now alive, in part, because their parents learned the truth about the impact of diet and lifestyle on their ability to be successful in pregnancy.

In my mind, I see some sort of mineral storehouse inside our bodies. In this storehouse there exist slots with labels for all the various vitamins, minerals, hormones, and such that our bodies need to function on a day-to-day basis. After all, it has a lot of work to make hundreds of thousands of new cells to replace the dying ones each day. It needs some raw materials. I see the storage areas as a large ice tray—the old-fashioned type you run the water over and watch each of the sections fill up. Once they are all full, you can place it into the freezer so it can do its job. Picture each of those ice tray slots with a different label for a certain nutrient we need. If your diet is deficient in certain items, then that slot will stay empty for a long time. This will cause, in some cases, big problems within the body.

Here is one example: anytime we consume an acid food (a food that creates or leaves an acid ash within our system may not necessarily have an extremely low pH when it enters the digestive system), our bodies must balance the ash to keep our overall pH within a safe range. One of the mechanisms for accomplishing this is by neutralizing acid with calcium. If the nutrient storehouse is low on calcium then the bones serve as a good resource for calcium. Thus, our system will borrow some calcium from the bones. Over a long period of time, this creates a disease called osteoporosis, which is a loss of bone density.

My mom suffered from osteoporosis for years prior to making significant diet changes. She has now been able to return her bone density back to the normal range. What happened? When she began to eat right, her nutrient storehouse was filled up, and she was able to begin paying back the bones for the calcium she had borrowed over the years.

Interestingly enough, dairy contains animal protein which leaves an acid ash. One of the big chants we hear for the promotion of dairy is that it contains supplemental calcium (which we evidently need for some reason…). The reality is that we need calcium to attempt to overcome the negative effects of an unhealthy, acid diet which is chiefly driven by the consumption of animal products. It seems to make sense to me that we can simply stop eating the things that cause or leave an acid ash, and along with that, stop the massive supplementation in an attempt to balance an unhealthy system overall.

The point with this as it relates to pregnancy is that it could be there is a mismatch in the necessary nutrients to either build a baby, or to even conceive to begin with. If your body is not fit to build a healthy baby, then maybe it has some failsafe to prevent pregnancy from even happening. This is just a theory, of course, but either way, the result is the same and filling up the nutrient storehouse makes a bunch of sense.

We have been through three fairly uneventful pregnancies. Well, pretty uneventful for me, that is. Nikki has a few words for me when I try to diminish her challenges of pregnancy. What I mean is that it seems like they were pretty much in alignment with about the smoothest possible pregnancies that one could have. Conception, when desired or attempted, was never a problem. Our kids are all pretty close to two years apart. Nikki supplemented with folic acid, B12, and a good prenatal vitamin just to be safe during each of the pregnancies. Our diet has continued to improve over the years, so Gabe, our oldest, would have gotten the muddiest ride in terms of Nikki's nutritional storehouse and ability, but he seems to be doing just fine. Nikki remains free of stretch marks of any kind.

We did keep up with regular doctor visits during the pregnancy with Gabe, but we also met with our doula regularly because she understood our lifestyle perspective. She walked us through the pregnancy and birthing process, teaching us along the way. This turned out to be a life-saver for us once the birthing began. With Farrell and Jake, we used a midwife and the same doula, so the regular visits were in a much more comfortable environment with people who really understood, appreciated, and agreed with our naturalistic approach to pregnancy.

The final trimester seems to stick out the most for each of us, especially the final month for each of them. For Gabe, we were not nearly as impatient, but for Farrell and then Jake, the last month seemed like an eternity. Nikki wanted the baby out and I just wanted whatever she wanted!

We greatly miss the child of one pregnancy that started unplanned and ended the same. We have always been excited about having a big family and so even though a fourth pregnancy was a surprise, it was a welcome one. About three months into it, we made a trip, as a family, on an airplane to attend a wedding. Had we known how that flight would impact the pregnancy, we certainly would not have taken it. During the visit, we lost the baby. We will never forget that trip. Nikki was in emotional pain immediately, but for some reason I tried to shrug it off. A few months had to pass before I really hurt for the situation. I hurt because I so love each of our kids that I wonder what another would have been like. Their personalities are so different from each other, and I feel that we lost something so precious that we can't even fathom it. Nothing can make it up or replace that baby. Secondly, I hurt because I was upset with myself for not grieving with Nikki, but instead became callous and distant to the whole situation. I love kids and I hope we have more, but I will always have a special spot for the one we lost. Thankfully, I know Jesus has a better special spot.

Birth

All of our kids were in the neighborhood of six pounds at birth. I remember as a kid that many of us were five or six pounds, and it was totally odd that we would hear of any newborn being more than eight pounds. That is the reason why I find it so interesting today that people think nothing of the fact that babies have gotten so much bigger. Is it just me or is it really obvious that the size of the baby has a direct relationship with the eating habits of the mom? I blame dairy products first, but I know that there are a lot of other contributing factors. Just plain overeating is a problem as well. Dairy is designed to take a relatively small calf, and make it into a full grown animal of hundreds of pounds. Clearly there is too much fat and too much of the wrong type of protein in it for it to be of any use to us as humans.

Gabe was born in a big regional hospital. He was carried full term, and the day the water broke our doula was there in a flash to help us. We stayed at home for the first few hours until we transitioned to the hospital. We opted against all drugs and equipment monitoring. When we arrived at the hospital, and infrequently thereafter, they checked to measure the dilation. Nikki was moving along well, but there was a problem that would halt progress for several hours. As Gabe's elongated head crowned, the problem was clear. The umbilical cord was wrapped around his neck, holding him back. After it was pulled over the top of his head, he popped right out.

The biggest challenges we faced with the birthing process had to do with the disrespect from the medical staff around our birthing plan. I was also amazed at the ambivalence of the doctor before and during the actual birth. I realize that this may have been her 10,000th birth, but it was a birth nonetheless and deserved to be treated as such. At one point, about an hour after Gabe was born (it was now about 1:30 am), I was confronted by a nurse, and then more boldly by the head nurse. The argument had to do with a vitamin K goop they wanted to put on his eyes.

The ointment contains an antibiotic medication which is designed as a safeguard from unknown, but potential, gonorrhea infection that could have been picked up in the birth canal. Babies are sometimes injected in the upper thigh with vitamin K due to low levels, and these eye drops or ointment is also commonplace. I was literally threatened by the head nurse that if I did not allow the application of this goop on Gabe's eyes, then we would not be allowed to take him home. As I think back, I wonder where he would have lived at the hospital if we were forced to leave without him…

The next day while Nikki was enjoying some time alone with him, one of the nurses came in and lambasted her for being such a terrible mom for preventing common modalities for her son. This was about the most hurtful thing anyone could have said to a first-time new mother already dealing with the natural effects of the post-birthing process. Needless to say, we saw enough to know future births would be different.

Farrell was born in Gabe's room on his bed. It worked well because the twin bed allowed for us to be around Nikki and have easy access to assist her. We had two wonderful mid-wives and our doula. The push time for labor was much less for Farrell. We took a walk down the street with Nikki which seemed to help. Sitting on the toilet was a comfortable place, along with a soak in the tub, but getting in and out of the tub was a bit of a pain.

Farrell was born without the amniotic sac breaking. This is technically called being "born in the caul." It is a very rare and healthy way of being born, because clearly the baby is protected during the entire birth process. It is odd to see a baby come out within the amniotic sac, however. It is also surprising how strong this sac is. We obviously did get her out of the sac and found out we had a beautiful little girl!

Interestingly enough, there is a medieval myth that babies who are born in the caul are free from the fear of ever dying by drowning. These babies could even sell this caul of protection to others (mainly sailors), and it was highly sought after, according to legend. I mention this because when Farrell was two, we were at a lodge near the border of Washington and Oregon. They happen to have an Olympic-sized pool, which our family enjoyed by ourselves. Jake was just a baby, so he stayed safely in his carrier. Both Gabe and Farrell needed our help to get around the pool because even the shallow end was too deep for them. Farrell got tired of this after a while and wanted out. In and out they both went, as it is with kids. They would run over and stick their feet in the hot tub, and then come running back. On one of these trips, I was near the center of the pool and Nikki was at the opposite end. Farrell thought she had suddenly gained dominance over the water and jumped right in without either of us seeing her. I must had heard her or seen it in the corner of my eye. I certainly never swam so fast and will never forget watching her flounder in and out of the water as I tried to get to her. When I did get to her she was still bobbing for air and may have taken a bit of water in but was ok and happy to be quickly lifted to the edge of the pool.

It doesn't end there. When she was four we were visiting eastern Washington for a go-kart race Gabe was in. The hotel we stayed in had a very small pool. I would estimate it was only fifteen feet by thirty feet. One evening, after a day at the race track, the pool area was packed and there must have been over twenty kids in the pool. I was in and out with Farrell, and with a push she was able to swim to the edge on her own from the center. At some point when Nikki and I were out of the pool, Farrell must have jumped into the center from the other side. I don't know how long it was before I noticed her, but once again I was on a rescue mission to save her! When I got her out her lips were slightly blue which was a little scary for all of us.

So much for the legend of the caul. Or, wait, maybe it is working!

Within an hour after Farrell was born, the house was cleaned up and cleared out, and we were sitting, holding our new little baby girl, watching a NASCAR race we had recorded. What a precious and special day.

Jake was also born at home. For him, we thought it would be interesting to attempt a water birth, so we planned for and rented a birthing tub and set it up in our living room. Nikki still has a thorn in her side about the fact that at some point she looked up and saw me "working" on my laptop while she was doing her thing in the pool. Truth be told (but she won't listen), I was searching for a web-based timer with a big graphic we could use. I did eventually find one (we are talking about three to five minutes of searching here, okay…), and was able to turn my laptop screen towards us so we could see the exact time Jake was born. Whew! I'm glad I finally got to air the truth around that.

Nikki's labor with Jake was similar to her labor with Farrell, and even shorter in length. We used all of the same methods other than including the birthing tub. The part we didn't know about was that it is actually better if I would have gotten in the tub with her and allowed her to sit on my thighs, creating a little canal between my legs for Jake to enter through. As an engineer (and after the fact of course), I have thought many times that a simple seat mechanism would be easy to design for this purpose although I would have been happy to get in with her. Anyway, you can probably guess that she had an extremely bruised and sore tailbone, which made the next few days the most uncomfortable of days after any of the births.

Jake was also nearly born in the caul, which by now we saw as a sign of good health. When his head crowned just seconds before he popped out, the sac broke all in one smooth motion. It was really neat to see all of this and how the water washed him up before he came up out of it for his first breath. Within an hour after he was born, we were once again back to a peaceful home. Nikki rested for a couple hours because of the soreness of her bum, but was up and about without hesitation after that.

Summary: Raising Healthy Kids

Raising healthy kids in an unhealthy, toxic world is quite a challenge. There is no perfection. That fact is an important reminder for me because I lean toward idealism in everything. Our kids are four, six, and eight years old this summer. We are learning as we go for sure. As we continue to improve and make changes in our choices and understanding, we implement new things for the family as a whole. The kids are quite literally learning with us. Our hope is that we give them the best opportunity possible to avoid many of the bad habits we picked up in our early years. In so doing, the unnatural within our culture will be natural for them and vice versa.

When they were babies, they had breast milk for about eighteen months each. As babies, they also got BarleyMax® on the pacifier until they were old enough to eat it dry off a spoon. If breast milk is not available, then the current recommendation by Hallelujah Acres is 1/3 equal amounts of the following: carrot juice, fresh organic goat's milk, and purified water.

Beyond that, and to keep this pretty simple, we basically just allowed their mouth maturity to determine what they were ready to eat. At a few months, they did not have teeth, but were able to mash soft fruit in their mouths. As their teeth came in, they could take progressively harder items. The thinking is that their entire digestive system develops at the same rate as their mouth and teeth. In other words, it may not be good to grind up a hard vegetable before they have teeth, because the rest of their digestive system may not be ready to handle this sort of item.

Today, the kids generally eat about the same as Nikki and I do. They, like all of us, waffle from liking one thing to refusing to eat it. However, the choices they have are always wide open in terms of the vast and broad overall healthy options for nourishment we have available to us. The quantities of food are somewhat self-determined but the items are the same for all.

CHAPTER FOURTEEN

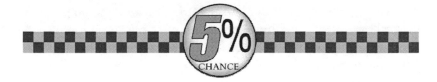

Creation Foundation

Food is a wonderful gift from God and a requirement to sustain life. God also uses our need for food to help us understand Him and our need for Him.

Sin happens, as I understand it, when we place something or someone in a position which is greater than God. It is common to hear someone say that Jesus was perfect. What He did was live a life free of sin. While He did so, He most certainly got some dirt between his toes. His life was not perfect in experience. He faced challenges and trials just as we do. It is important to understand that the perfection and idealism that we seek is often sinful because we attempt to circumvent the need for God by controlling the environment into our form of perfection. These efforts are futile and ultimately impossible in and of themselves. Jesus is successful in permanently seating Father God as the chief focus of His worship. Jesus has never faltered in this. That is the sort of perfection He has achieved and what we should seek.

What does all this have to do with our food? Well, it is actually closely tied to our love of food, which is actually worship of food and is called gluttony.

Gluttony is a sin and it is mentioned many times in the Bible. It is not, however, considered a sin universally. Depending upon the culture it could be seen as either a vice or a status symbol. The relative affluence of the culture affects this view in both ways. The wealthy may take pride in the security of having plenty, and may be prone to show it off, but may be faced with the results of social backlash when confronted with view of the less fortunate.

Gluttony according to Wikipedia:

"Gluttony, derived from the Latin gluttire, meaning to gulp down or swallow, means over-indulgence and over-consumption of food, drink, or intoxicants to the point of waste. In some Christian denominations, it is considered one of the seven deadly sins—a misplaced desire of food or its withholding from the needy."

What I think of when I read that is, at what point do I reach the line of acceptable indulgence? After all, we want to know when we have crossed over it, right? Furthermore, it perplexes me to think we can't go out and have a nice meal with family, and enjoy eating whatever we want in as much quantity as we would like. My take on this is that for the most part, we should attempt to live according to our needs, and occasionally we should feel comfortable with a bit of indulgence, provided it does not harm ourselves or others. So how does that play out in my life? I don't live for food. Food is a tool. But, there are some meals, times and social events which are simply wonderful, divine, and nearly indescribable and these often revolve around or are engulfed in food. I believe we should enjoy these times and remain very reasonable about our consumption on a day-to-day basis.

I want to begin by simply laying a foundation that food is not a sin, yet gluttony is. Because of my own propensities around the word "sin," I feel better about describing it. If you are not a

Christian and the word "sin" feels condemning then let me explain a bit further.

All Christians are sinners because we allow created things to be elevated above the Creator God. The foundation of sin is simply worshiping something above God. The vernacular used by Christians to describe the non-Christian is "the lost". Regardless of our cleanliness outwardly, inwardly (spiritually) we are broken and hemorrhaging in pain. We search endlessly for answers to our pain until such time as we are saved or become exhausted. Adversity propels us to begin searching anew. The source of our pain is our separation from our Creator. Jesus is the Savior because He enables reconciliation to our Creator God.

So, the lost can make the same choices as the saved yet not see the result as sin (i.e. being a sinner). We must first realize our lostness, then our need for answers and finally the sufficiency of Jesus as savior before we can rightly see our offenses as sin.

This is important because many followers of Christ would admit that gluttony is a pervasive sin. It would be difficult to find even one among the saved and the lost who has not succumbed to the taunts of gluttony. Gluttony can manifest in many forms inside and outside of the context of food. Here are some examples of how it comes to life as it threatens our relationship with God and those around us:

> **Impatience**. Eating before it is time or never letting yourself feel a bit of hunger. This is solely out of habit and due to the pleasing of the palate or physical self, and is contrary to what we know and believe about where our full satisfaction should come from. I feel best on an empty stomach or with a slight ache for some nourishment. As a culture we fear this place and so we stay far from it.

> **I Deserve The Best**. We see delicacies and enormous flavors. The birth of excitotoxins is the solution for our endless yearning for more flavor, more taste, more and more. We see shows of people who travel the world looking for, tasting, and taking pleasure from the very

best of foods. It is not that we should seem to deprive ourselves of our wonderful God-given and nourishing foods, but the never-satisfied palate is dangerous.

Additions or Stimulants. Similar to any addictive draw, food is one that brings pleasures mentally and physically. There are literally hundreds of unnatural flavorings that are used in food or sold as a seasoning in an attempt to fulfill this desire. Dr. Russell Blaylock explains excitotoxins, the role they play in food, and the diseases they are contributing towards in his book entitled Excitotoxins.

Seconds Please. We have a restaurant near us called The Claim Jumper. They have good quality food, but their claim to fame socially is the size of their plates. Our family of five could easily feed from a single plate, yet it is common to see each person order their own and do a decent job of clearing it. We find comfort in a full table, belly, or bank account instead of in God. Quantity is one of the easiest forms of gluttony to grasp. We all have a voracious appetite for more.

Live To Eat. We tend to approach food with an excessive desire. We get very excited about eating and the prospect of food. We rarely meet for the sake of meeting, but more commonly for the excuse of eating. We are simply too eager for our next meal. I have a friend who told a story of how his father always talked about the contents of the next meal before the current one was complete.

Food is fun and should be enjoyed, but it is clear from these items that we take it where it is not intended to go. Why is the gluttony of food so pervasive?

A friend recently helped me to understand this more clearly. He is a self diagnosed "gluttoner", overweight and burdened with the results physically, mentally, and spiritually of his choices on a daily basis. While we were catching up recently, he asked if I knew why gluttony was so difficult to overcome. Of course I was all ears. What he described made sense and came from a perspective I had not ever realized prior to that conversation.

It is expected that in close-knit Christian relationships we will talk about the struggles we face in socially unacceptable sins. Sexual sins bubble to the top. It isn't as common that we address or face the socially acceptable sins. For example, the way we use our time, money, or food. Last I checked however, a sin is a sin and does the same work of removing Jesus from the top seat in our list of idols.

My friend pointed out that we can easily coach someone close to us about the negative effects of pornography. Or, if he has a problem with drinking or lust, then these too are like a bad route to work—some routes should simply be avoided altogether.

Food, on the other hand, is a different challenge because we can't just avoid food altogether. In fact, it may be the only really common tool we cannot and should not avoid all together that leads the majority of us, if not all of us, into inappropriate worship (of the food).

If all of this talk of gluttony just seems over the top then set aside your food for a few days and limit yourself to just fresh raw vegetables and fruit or juice from either or both. If you can do that for a few days and not have any negative effects then maybe you are one of the three people on the planet that don't have a problem with gluttony.

As I think through this, I realize how really impossible the task before us is in our own strength. At the same time, I am all the more thankful God lives in us to guide and provide the ultimate comfort.

> In Proverbs 23:1-2 we read, "When you sit to eat with a ruler, observe carefully what is before you, and put a knife to your throat if you are given to appetite (gluttony)."

The warning here is similar to many throughout the Bible where we are warned to worship God above everything else. The idea of putting a knife to the throat simply indicates the severity of worshiping food, comfort, wealth, etc. above God. If you have a Bible handy, flip to Proverbs 23 and read all of it. I hope you see there is some good wisdom for our dietary choices, but more so there is a deeper message and truth contained within. To figure this out, ask yourself why God requires us, by design, to need food? Like many similar questions you could ponder, you will quickly get to a common answer.

Pay special attention to Proverbs 23:20-21 where we see a strong warning:

> "Be not among drunkards or among gluttonous eaters of meat, for the drunkard and the glutton will come to poverty, and slumber will clothe them with rags."

In Paul's letter to the church of Philippi (Philippians 3:17-21) he wrote,

> "Brothers, join in imitating me, and keep your eyes on those who walk according to the example you have in us. For many, of whom I have often told you and now tell you even with tears, walk as enemies of the cross of Christ. Their end is destruction, their god is their belly, and they glory in their shame, with minds set on earthly things. But our citizenship is in heaven, and from it we await a Savior, the Lord Jesus Christ, who will transform our lowly body to be like His glorious body, by the power that enables Him even to subject all things to Himself."

We are taught to be "like Christ" when in reality none of us will ever be anything like Christ at all. He lived a life free of sin (meaning that He never worshiped anything above His Father, God), He gave Himself for us, He redeems us daily through His work on the cross, and He comforts us with His mighty and careful hand.

What we should attempt is to imitate Christ. We should seek to worship as He worshiped. We tend to worship created things instead of the Creator God. Food is a tool provided by the Creator. Food is part of this creation. It is not the Creator and should not be worshiped in any form or manner. We will achieve success in worship as Christ did to the extent that we can allow Jesus to be most highly exalted followed by our spouse, and everything else somewhere below that. It is possible. It may be momentary and may seem like a never-ending challenge, but it is most certainly possible.

The most important thing I have found in being able to successfully worship God in and through all things is not a stoic focus on that thing as some may assume. There is, I think, a much simpler path but it is not one that would be stumbled across without some forethought. What seems to be most important is to understand our identity in Christ properly. Once we accomplish this, then we are able to respond properly to many things in life instead of the obvious approach, which may look a lot like box checking or self-discipline. I am an engineer so I tend to have fairly square corners. I like accuracy and strive for perfection – even though I am learning perfection is a myth. Therefore, I tend to lean towards the attempt at self-discipline instead of simply recognizing who I am.

So, who are we? I mean, if we are Christians, what does that mean and how does that understanding transform us on a moment-by-moment basis through our days? How can we capture success in our diet by understanding who we are in Christ?

At the core, being in Christ means that everything is about who we are rather than what we do. Clearly, this understanding enables complete freedom from shame, fear and worry (Romans 6:14-15). We recognize our position in Christ through the obedience of baptism. In it we experience a spiritual death, burial and resurrection. Many people talk about eternal life as a destiny when, in reality, it is a process that has already begun since we are in Christ. Nothing we have done or can do has any impact on our true identity. Our efforts in this matter would be like trying to dry a single spot on our body while we were under water – it would be a waste of time. We are new because of redemption through Jesus. Most of us, at some point during our lives, realize we are redeemed (in Christ) and we finally accept the reality. From that point, it is important that we continue on and seek to more fully understand the gift. We do this through education, and in so doing, we become fully aware of our true identity (Heb. 5:11-14).

I previously asked why God made us to need food. He could quite easily have designed us to not require food. We could somehow take in energy and nutrients some other way. But for some reason, He inserted the necessity of food consumption. Or, was it just a necessity? I really enjoy food so maybe He did it for our joy. It was probably for both reasons because our joy leads to His glorification. I was recently day-dreaming about this topic while driving and I thought about something interesting.

To begin with, the traditional five senses are sight, hearing, touch, smell and taste. What would you eat if you could not taste anything? Seriously, what would you eat? I think I would choose something that felt good in my mouth, or maybe something that smelled good as I was eating it. Maybe I'd choose something that simply looked divine. Well, what if we took away taste and smell? Now all you could do is look at the food, feel it going down, and I guess, listen to whatever it sounds like to eat it or prepare it.

If we allow enough time to pass, and we follow this line of thinking far enough, we will find that we would be eating the thing that cost the least. We have food manufacturers filled with talented people today that are forced to work within the bounds of our senses as they attempt to create irresistible products. Their jobs would be so much easier if all they had to do was create a thing that looked wonderful, didn't kill us instantly and was super cheap!

This still doesn't answer the question of why God created us to need food. I think that it is fairly straight forward and similar to many other experiences that He creates for us in life. He first wants us to enjoy our food (and of course through that we can also glorify Him), giving Him the credit for our joy in food. God was wise in developing His requirement for us to need food and the integrating of that need with our senses. This prevents us from eating junk that would quickly render us dead. Also, it allows us to glorify and worship Him as we bite into and enjoy a juicy sweet organic red pepper.

Don't Mess With My Food

Is it now a bit clearer why most Christians avoid the discussion of the gluttony of food? It is common to hear a teacher mention food in a list of sins that we adopt for our own, but rarely will they dig any deeper. The truth is that they simply don't know very much about gluttony using food, and they are most likely just as deep into it as those they are charged to lead. Furthermore, this isn't really the proper role for a teaching pastor, because their emphasis should be on teaching Jesus. The point is that, if we can keep our focus on the one, true God, then none of the rest of this matters. It will just simply sort of fix itself and go away.

In Matthew 6:31-33 we read about this very thing.

> "Therefore do not be anxious, saying, 'What shall we eat?' or 'What shall we drink?' or 'What shall we wear?' For the Gentiles seek after all these things, and your heavenly Father knows that you need them all. But seek first the kingdom of God and His righteousness, and all these things will be added to you."

Isn't it wonderful to see how simple these concepts are to understand when they are made clear? I always dreamed about a cool car being "added to me." Now I realize what is added to me is everything I need to sustain a full and joyful life—quite literally by simply seeking God first. My seeking of Him works itself out tangibly through my understanding of my identity in Him – knowing who I am.

Like many other quality teachings that happen within the church body, some focus should be invested and promoted in the area of gluttony of food. It is clearly a piece of the message God has for us, and there are plenty of Christians equipped with the ability to educate others in this area. Unfortunately, there are an enormous number of people that are stricken with the results of not understanding in this area. The prayer lists are filled with the results of ignorance in the area of gluttony.

Occasionally I get threatening emails, phone calls, voice mails and letters. People will criticize my perspective in their blogs, on the news, in print or other forms. One of the most recent threats I got via voice mail indicated, using the most choice of words, that my position on health care (which, by the way, should be called "disease care") was wrong. I wonder if this person has spent a quarter of their life learning, studying, and putting into practice for the purpose of healing, education, and leadership the truths about diet, lifestyle, and the impact these have on our health? As I listened to the voice mail, two things came to mind that if I had a few minutes with the sender at a time when he was really willing to listen, it would most certainly change his perspective on the topic forever.

The two things are: a) forcing companies to pay for disease care will drive salaries down in an equal proportion, and, b) telling entrepreneurs how to spend their profits will kill the entire free market system that our country thrives upon. If you want to discuss more, then find me.

Another time, an employee literally got in my face, and was yelling at me and accusing me of heresy because of my teaching in the area of nutrition. I got the smattering of saliva with the finger in my chest while Scriptures were flying. I feel bad for this person to this day. I hurt for him because he is so ignorant of the bigger truth that is so much greater and deeper than anything to do with food. I intend for my worship to be of Jesus, and I hope and pray for the same for him and you. If, because I am writing a book on the relationship between lifestyle choices and disease, it seems as if the topic of food is most important to me, then please let me set the record straight.

I love food. I enjoy food. I take great pleasure in playing in the kitchen, but I ultimately see food as a tool. It is a necessary tool for me to continue to serve and worship the only true God, who is Jesus Christ. The church I attend is all about Jesus, and I am proud to admit my membership to this social group that is culturally liberal and doctrinally conservative. Under this tutelage and the leading the Holy Spirit, I have grown greatly. You, too, can enjoy some of the teaching as a supplement to the local group of Christians whom you worship with and do life with. If you're curious, you can learn more about the church I attend, Mars Hill Church, at www.marshillchurch.org.

To wrap this section up, I want to be clear that food is not a sin, but what we do with our food, and our desire and worship of food, can be and in many cases is a sin. So, please don't send me an email asking me if you should repent of eating a burger!

Original Intent

What did God really intend when He created man? What happened that may have changed or impacted His plan—or was His plan really changed? If there was an initial or an original plan and we have strayed from it, is there a return to it? If so, when?

As I get older, I have more and more respect for those current and past who challenged their brains with deep questions. It seems many of us choose to consume life without questions, rather than living life by questioning. To be clear, I have never considered myself to be much of a thinker (i.e. smart), but I do like to question things and then dig for answers. I have added a lot of color to my life using this approach, and I know I am light years closer to knowing truth in various areas because I question, question, question until I feel I understand the real answers. I suppose I am a bit like Josh, played by Tom Hanks and David Moscow, in the movie Big (1988) when he commented, while in conference with colleagues of the toy company he worked at, regarding his inability to understand. He simply says, "I don't get it" as they bantered a marketing scheme for a toy that he didn't think would be the least bit interesting to kids. The key is that he stood up and said he didn't understand something.

This brings me to a big question I am going to challenge you with—and then, since this is my book, I will give you my answers to ponder. If you can't add to them or take away from them then find another question to dig upon.

What is the meaning of life? Don't stop reading, I will make this quick. You will be better off for it and like a good trial lawyer, I will tie this all back together soon.

What is the meaning of life? Have you ever thought about it? I mean for more than seven seconds until something less taxing hits your brain. Get a yellow note pad out and write down a question, then just begin making notes about what comes to mind. Or, if you want a quick answer based on someone else's yellow note pad time, just Google, Bing, or Wikipedia the question…

Why I think I am here: *Glorify by expressing His joy daily and sharing it with others.*

There is a lot more to this, of course, but the main points are as follows. God is made up of a three entities, God, Jesus, and the Holy Spirit. Each of these exists in the one God, and They have existed since before They decided to create us and the world. I respect and love God by knowing Him, believing Him, trusting Him, and respecting Him. God is sovereign over all, which means He is in all, through all, and part of all. This is the reason why there are so many holy wars, because people who are led to follow false gods get angry when they learn that the one real God says He stands over everything, including their god. Jesus was a gift for us because He enabled us to live free of our own junk. He granted us redemption. He allowed Himself to be the ultimate sacrifice for us so we don't have to carry the liability of our own actions from an eternal perspective. That means we don't have to worry about our eternal lives because Jesus has taken care of it, but it does not magically protect us from the ramifications of our own decisions. The Holy Spirit is a gift in Himself. He is the manifestation of God in and through us. God is sovereign through the Holy Spirit.

That gives you the basic framework for my answer to the meaning of life. Now, let me explain how all that ties into what I eat.

If I am to know Him, love Him, and truly live out the joy He intends for me, can I best do that through proper or improper treatment of my physical body? You see, every one of our decisions in life is thrown over to our subconscious where a decision is made based on what we truly believe life is about. It's based on what our world view is, so to speak. Depending upon what we believe—not what we say we believe, but what we truly believe—drives every one of our actions and decisions. Therefore, it is first important to know what you believe. Again, not what you say you believe with your mouth, but what you truly believe. If you don't know then just look back at your choices and that will be an invaluable indication of what you believe in your heart. If you do look, and you don't like what you see, then you are on a wonderful new path of determining how you change what you truly believe into what you really want to believe. That is one of life's biggest challenges, and sadly only very few stand on the question long enough to figure it out. I hope you enjoy this adventure. That is what He intends.

I am not fun to be around when I am not feeling well. It has been years since anyone has had to deal with this, but I remember days long ago when I could be demanding and just plain difficult if I didn't feel well. Eating right, getting good sleep, exercising regularly, mitigating stress, and managing my priorities to ensure the important things get the top spots all contribute to me truly living what I believe to be truth. The times when I don't make the right choice in these areas, I realize I am taking something away from myself and my family and friends.

I also realize each of us gets caught up in living our story (self-worship). We are so funny in the things we do. We sit in a circle and talk about our struggles or our blessings, and then after a good long discussion, we agree to bow our heads and talk mainly about the same things, this time including God. Was God not listening the first time? Prayer is chiefly for us in the context in which we do it. Prayer should actually be a part of our worship, and if we saw it in this way, the result of our prayers would sound and look much different. The key here is to make a dynamic shift from self-worship to God-worship. We need to stop living out our story while asking God to be a part of it. And, we need to begin living as if we are blessed to be a part, a scene, within His great big epic story. We don't ask Him to come and join us, help us, save us, protect us in the midst of our story. We do realize the great honor of being part of His magnificent and wonderful story. When we are successful in accomplishing this, then we get the gift of His true joy through anything we face.

Living as healthy of a lifestyle as possible enables me to focus on God and not myself. That is not to say living and eating healthy is a magic pill for a tighter relationship with God. I do believe I notice an additional clarity of mind and seemingly clearer access to God when I am healthy, but that should not be a surprise. If my body is in shape and not feeling this or that, then I am less likely to actually be thinking about it. If I am not thinking about it, then I am less likely to be worshiping it.

Scriptural References
In the rest of this chapter, I have invested in reviewing Scripture that either supports or seemingly distorts the constitution of our Creator's intent for us physically.

Since God started "In the beginning...", I will follow His lead.

In Genesis 1:29, God clearly gives some guidance and direction to His perfect creation for how they should nourish their physical bodies.

> *"And God said, Behold, I have given you every plant yielding seed that is on the face of all the earth, and every tree with seed in its fruit. You shall have them for food."*

It is also important as you look through these Scriptures and this entire concept, if you are a believer in God, to watch for parallels of truth with His story. He never contradicts Himself, and I have seen countless patterns in my life that ultimately lead to a deeper faith and a stronger belief in a certain direction because I realized this connection. In this case, God is giving us direction on how to nourish our physical body. Would it not make sense that He would also give us indication as to how we are to be nourished spiritually?

In John 6:47-51 we read Jesus' words regarding our spiritual nourishment,

> *"I tell you the truth, anyone who believes has eternal life. Yes, I am the bread of life! Your ancestors ate manna in the wilderness, but they all died. Anyone who eats the bread from heaven, however, will never die. I am the living bread that came down from heaven. Anyone who eats this bread will live forever; and this bread, which I will offer so the world may live, is my flesh."*

In the years that I have been studying and practicing on the laboratory of one (myself), I have seen countless ways in which I can draw correlation between what I now know to be truth regarding how we are to live physically with how we are to live spiritually.

Scripture can also be confusing because we don't fully understand the context or the purpose therein. In Ezekiel chapter 34, we see something very interesting, and potentially confusing. It is clear the chapter is talking about the ultimate Savior, Jesus, and what He will do for God's children. But, it is also talking about the Israelites and what He has planned for them in shorter terms. Read verse 10 and notice it indicates that the shepherds were actually consuming or eating the flock. Does that mean that the Israelite leaders were eating the people that they were leading? No, it is a metaphoric association of actual sheep and shepherds. The reference to the shepherds eating the flock could not accurately be assumed to mean that the leaders of the people actually ate the people. I mention this because there are many more things in the Bible that we do not understand (generally) than those that we do. The book is quite literally the Word of God. It is God manifest in our lives. It is real, true and at least three-dimensional.

Animal Sacrifice

Animal sacrifice was instituted by God with the indication that there must be a blood sacrifice in exchange for our fall. In the grand story, Jesus served as the ultimate sacrifice. He paid the ultimate price for each of us, thus there is no need for animal sacrifice post His death and resurrection.

The connection we need to see here is that at a point in history, God required animal sacrifice (due to Adam and Eve eating the forbidden fruit in the Garden of Eden—this is known as the Fall of Man). At a point later in history, God allowed the consumption of animal flesh in association with the sacrifice. The sacrifice was purposed for atonement for us falling short (regularly). The consumption of the animal products is at least in part negated if the sacrifice itself is no longer needed.

Additionally, about the same time (Genesis 6:3), God limited the life span of man to 120 years. Previously, many people lived in excess of 900 years. There are no other environmental or noteworthy changes as to why life was limited to this seemingly short time frame. Did the flood change the earth in some way to make it more toxic? Did something happen with the air that causes us to age more quickly? Does it have something to do with the sun or sun exposure? Could it be that something as simple as eating animal products and the negative effects of such consumption could single-handedly reduce the life expectancy by nearly 90% in just a few generations? I don't believe the consumption of meat is the only factor, but it certainly is a significant contributor.

"UNCLE"

After reading this far, and especially if this is your first introduction to this information, you may be about to cry out "uncle" as if to say you give up and you want the pain to stop. Interestingly enough, there is actually a reason for the pain. That will the case for some but for others, this book is a breath of fresh air. However, you may be wondering why God allowed you to face what you've had to physically. As with everything, never doubt that there is a plan and a purpose that is much greater than our scene in God's great big story. Listen up, because I know you are going to enjoy this colossal nugget.

Do you ever wonder why life is so tough and what the point of all the difficulties is? If it is that we lack knowledge, wisdom or understanding, could not our all-knowing, all-loving, all-powerful God just simply inject this knowledge into us somehow?

Obviously there are several problems with this, starting with the fact we all know, that love would not and could not exist if we did not have the ability to choose. And it is often the result of our choices that bring about the challenges we face. Although we have no choice about our salvation (Romans 8), we do have some choice over the few years we live here on earth. The sole purpose for this choice is so we may understand and share in love, chiefly in the love of God by loving Him and by experiencing His love.

As I write this book, there are many people struggling financially. I have learned that this, like everything, is either initiated or authorized by God. As you know, we are built to soar as eagles in our endeavors with God. The problem is that we often like to soar without Him if everything goes really well. In other words, we need adversity to realize our true need for God. Sometimes this adversity comes individually or in pockets. Other times, it comes to a people group, a country, or even comes globally. Here are some examples cited by John Piper.

- God promises the heir when Abraham and Sarah are too old to have children.
- God splits the Red Sea when Israel is hopelessly trapped by Pharaoh's army.
- God gives manna when there is no food in the wilderness.
- God stops the Jordan River when it's time to take the land.
- When a city stands in the way, God makes the walls fall down.
- When the Midianites were as many as the sand of the sea, God whittled Gideon's army down to 300 so God would get the glory for the victory.
- When Goliath defies the armies of the Lord, God sends a boy with a sling and five stones.
- When the Son of God is to come into the world, God calls a virgin to conceive.
- And when the mighty devil himself is to be defeated, a Lamb goes to the slaughter.

We can all cite times when terrible things that don't make sense have happened to people, or when it seems like God did not show up in the nick of time to save someone, something, or a group of people. I know this, too, is part of His master plan.

God does in fact use adversity, but why? With more help from John Piper, here are some reasons:

- To expose hidden sin and to bring us to repentance and cleansing.
- To wake us up to the constant and desperate condition of the developing world where there is always and only recession of the worst kind.

- To relocate the roots of our joy in His grace rather than in our goods, in His mercy rather than our money, and in His worth rather than our wealth.

- To advance His saving mission in the world—the spread of the gospel and the growth of His Church—precisely at a time when human resources are least able to support it, thus guarding His glory.

- He intends for the Church to care for its hurting members and to grow in the gift of love.

I further believe there are various different kinds of adversity that God may use to accomplish His will through us. It is sort of like He is saying that He has given us some choice, but that He is also going to create a clear path and will provide some adversity if we wander, in an effort to get us back to His path, plan and will. If you read Romans 12:2, you will see that our lives will be filled with adversity by the very nature of the fact that we live with the results of living based on the "patterns of this world." That very adversity can and is used by God to draw us to Himself.

There are also other forms of adversity, like the following, for example:

- Communication
- Physical ailment
- Pride and selfishness
- Danger and fear
- Persecution and Strain

Again, you are likely wondering what this has to do with food, diet, and our physical health, right? Think of each of these forms of adversity sitting in front of you on the table as a Rubik's Cube. So you have five Rubik's Cubes sitting in front of you and they are all messed up. Well, actually they may not all be messed up— you may have mastered one or more of them. And, as you read along, you will see that this is the point!

In this case, let's pick on Rev. George Malkmus. I know that he, by God's grace, has pretty much fixed the Rubik's Cube that is marked with "physical ailment." God has shown him the clear path to how and why physical ailments happen, thus understanding how to prevent it becomes fairly straightforward. The pattern of living required to keep this Rubik's Cube with all the colors on matching sides, however, is a daily challenge—even for Rev. Malkmus.

Now, what about the other four cubes? Could any of us master all of them, all the time? Furthermore, if we did master them, would we be free of adversity? I believe we can master them, and I believe we can live a life free of adversity. In fact, by so doing, we have basically described the state of living we will experience once we are eternally glorified. We will be free of adversity and the bondage of this world. We will be able to live in a state of perfection!

Am I saying a man or woman can live perfectly? No, but what I am saying is that through a life of testing, trials, and lots of adversity, we can master the five forms of adversity. But, by so doing, we spend our lives with God. We share our space with the Holy Spirit daily. Jesus intercedes for us, and the Father protects and provides for us. Once we spend forty, fifty, or ninety years working on this with God, we quite literally spend our lives in communion with Him. Once we are successful in knowing Him, then we no longer need the adversity nor does it bother us if it remains. Remember what the purpose of the adversity is—to draw us to Himself.

If the idea of making changes in your diet and lifestyle cause you some discomfort, then please take additional comfort in knowing the source and purpose of this adversity that is holy, ordained, and acceptable to God. He loves each of us enough to create multiple pathways for us to experience His joy as we let go of our plan and grab on to His.

Are You A Christian?

I would be deeply discouraged if you applied all the health related principles of this book and lived a long, fruitful life, while at the same time remained lost or separated from our God. If this is your case, God's good news (gospel) is that the Lord Jesus Christ is our redeemer. By placing our faith and trust in Him alone, we are saved, and gain a new identity in Christ. If you have not, will you place your faith in Christ now? If you will, please write to me, and I will send you a Bible and other helpful information. It would mean more to me to hear this news from only you than to help millions of people find physical healing alone.

In Luke 5:17-26, we see this pattern lived out by Jesus. He is presented with a paralyzed man whose friends were so bold as to lower him through the roof of the building where Jesus was speaking and surrounded by a crowd so that Jesus may heal their friend. Jesus first said, "Man, your sins are forgiven you." He then explained to the crowd that He had authority to forgive sin. Jesus finished by healing the man physically, "I say to you, rise, pick up your bed and go home." Jesus' main concern is for our hearts to be reconciled to God and He demonstrated that in the order of events described here.

CHAPTER FIFTEEN

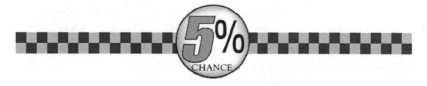

Fasting & Feasting

I was recently asked about the Daniel Fast, which is also known as the Daniel Diet. My initial reaction is simple. "If in ten days, I can look noticeably better, then that is certainly something that deserves a bit more attention." Here is a slightly deeper analysis.

Daniel 1:8-16

1) What is the purpose of a "fast?"
Fasting is, biblically speaking, a time for us to get our eyes off of the things of this world and onto God. We could fast from lots of things in our culture, but most tend to think of food when fasting. We could also, without feeling hypocritical, choose to "fast" for physical reasons. The purpose for this fast is generally to rest the body's digestive system and allow cleansing. Some people do this annually for a month or so. I agree that it is a healthy approach, but would not endorse water fasting since the detoxification is often severe and can be dangerous. Fresh juice

fasting, or even raw food fasting is a great way for people who are entrenched in the standard American diet to clean themselves up for a period of time. More on that below...

2) Live the truth... temporarily?

If you go all the way back to creation and ignore what happened after sin entered the world, you will quickly see what God's "original intent" was for our physical health, healing, and wholeness. He intended us to eat raw produce! Read Genesis 1:29 for His specific assignment in this regard. So, here is the thing. I believe we should eat as much raw, organic produce as we can, all the time. At the same time, given the data we have from the research done by doctors like Dr. Colin Campbell on those who consume animal products, chemically-filled processed foods, and such, it seems to make sense to limit or even eliminate those from our family regimes. Doing a cleansing fast for a period of time each year, in my opinion, is worse for your physical body than just eating a more balanced diet all the time, which contains a majority percentage of raw, organic produce. The ups and downs in your system can be difficult and the mental part is deceiving.

By cleansing for a few weeks a year, we give way to the thinking that we can just eat anything we want the rest of the year until as the time of the cleansing comes around again and we "sacrifice" for a few weeks. A few bites here, a few pounds there, oh, don't worry, the cleanse will clear it up. Furthermore, we really miss the benefits of living a healthy lifestyle. I was healed of cancer, my wife of irritable bowel syndrome (IBS), and our kids have generally been free of sickness their entire lives. That is not to say there isn't a rare occasion of some bug that comes around, but it is very infrequent, minor in terms of symptoms, never requires a doctor's visit, and it is uncommon that we even use any sort of medicine other than a mild pacifier.

In addition, my family's physical bodies are fit and healthy. We feel good about ourselves. Others regularly comment on the beauty of our family. Some stare in astonishment when they see full plates of salads and veggies for our kids.

So my encouragement to you would be to look at this as a journey. I would suggest a nice steady growth pattern starting right where you are would be a great trajectory. Don't feel like you need to conquer the world this week. Now, with that you need to demonstrate something that is uncommon in our culture. That is self-discipline and a box of commitment. You need to continue to educate your mind and pray for revelation and strength to stay on track. Not making a massive change in the beginning means you need to walk a slight upslope forever. Yes, forever. Think about it. A big change now means that inevitably you will walk a down-slope for the next couple of years back to where you are. Doesn't it make more sense to just start where you are, commit to the journey and begin making changes? You can do it! I know you can.

3) The veggie/vegan argument - biblically speaking...

I am often asked why I am a vegan Christian. The thing that people get confused on is that they think I or anyone else is saying that eating this or that is a sin. That would be wrong. All I am saying is that God's clear original intent was for us to be raw vegans. Getting sick wasn't His intent either, and although from a grand perspective sickness is because of sin, it is not because of the individual sin (i.e. do something wrong, eat the wrong thing = get sick). It just isn't so. Sickness is because of the fall of man (i.e., man sinned therefore we are all forced to live in an imperfect world where we need the redemptive blessing of Jesus Christ). With that, we have the free choice to avoid certain foods that are known to cause things like disease and sickness. If someone wants to reduce their chances of getting cancer or heart disease, they can easily make some lifestyle choices that would enable them to do that. If a spouse wants to be in shape and present their body to their husband or wife and to God in perfect shape, then the diet and lifestyle choices they need to make are fairly straightforward. If a driver wants to avoid getting a speeding ticket, then they had better not speed, right?

So the idea here is that it is not a sin to eat this or that, but the original intent of God was for us to be a raw vegan (before sin entered the world), and it is our own choice to live a lifestyle that is honoring to Him and the gift of life He gave us. Read Romans 12, Genesis 1:29, Corinthians 10:31. I think Romans 14:2-3 is comical. It does require more faith to eat meat because I know it will kill me!

Another common term you may hear is "feasting." It is used by some to avoid the word fasting, but it may mean the same thing. It is also used by some to describe how they feel about their food. Fasting seems to have a negative connotation while feasting is more positive and reeks of abundance. I have done a forty day "green coconut feast." There was nothing spiritual about this, per se. I just wanted to experience a lot of greens and see the impact in my life. I didn't eat just green coconuts, by the way. I ate all things green along with as much coconut as I wanted! It truly was a feast, and it was fun to be able to experiment with various different ingredients.

CHAPTER SIXTEEN

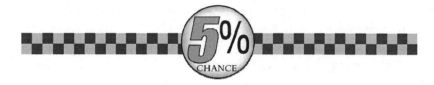

The Facts

We were created to live healthfully for a long time on limited raw, fresh, organic, vine-ripened produce. We also have the physical ability to sustain ourselves with much less variety than we often think we require. In India, where most of the mangos are grown, one could enjoy (or not enjoy, depending upon your preference) a period through the year where you could quite literally eat as much and as many mangos as you want and not begin to make a dent in the resource. The nutrients that come from a particular plant are not altogether unique. Sure, some produce contains increased or decreased amounts of certain nutrients, but it is possible to sustain life on very few of these life-giving nutrients. We see it lived out everyday as people gorge themselves on substances they call food, yet ones that are totally devoid of any nutritional value. Somehow, our bodies are able to maintain themselves even while we provide only little or no high quality, living nutrients.

The majority of the produce on earth dies on the vine. Most of it is never picked, or even looked upon. It will grow and die and the cycle continues. At our office, we have some blackberry bushes near one side of the parking lot. There are thousands of berries on them each year, and I think my kids and I are the only ones who actually eat any of them. We make such a small dent that it is difficult to imagine how many people could actually be enjoying this wonderful fruit. I searched and searched for some facts on how much or what percentage of the world is deficient in food sources, specifically the areas that are deprived of the sufficient supply of food to sustain healthy life. You can quickly begin to see the connection that I want to bridge here. Clearly, the answer for our food shortage problem is to redefine what food is. Could it be that the redefinition of food has already happened and we are relying on a false definition, which is currently causing the shortage in supply? Well, maybe not. It could be that we just have a distribution or logistical problem, but I would venture to guess that we do have a definition problem. If we redefine food back to what it is supposed to be, then we can focus on the simple task of distributing that food. We can also educate others on how to produce food throughout the world and literally solve the hunger and shortages quickly.

We have expanded our view of the definition of food, and then we have applied inappropriate focus on things that should not be considered food. At the same time, we have ignored the real food that is simply dying on the vine.

Based on this brief analysis, I believe we have more than enough food to supply everyone's needs many times over. The problem could easily be solved through first narrowing our definition of food, and then implementing a distribution system to ensure proper and necessary movement of the real food.

A couple of years ago, I set out to help my kids with a little school project. I thought it would be neat to build a little mobile that showed a couple of planets and how they revolved around each other. I wanted to do something extra special with Earth.

My plan was to add a little wire that would spin around Earth, which would be in position to indicate the thickness of the atmosphere. This would be a great demonstration which would show the actual size of the livable area around Earth.

What I wanted to show was how thick (or thin) the atmosphere is. I thought this would be interesting mainly because I look out at the space and size of the universe, dream about the unknown galaxies, and quite literally live in amazement of the size of creation! When you consider that vast size, the space in which we live, which was specially and specifically designed for us to sustain life, has more meaning. I wanted to build this little model so it would enable my kids to see how really small that space was that God created for us to sustain life. What I found still shocks me to think about to this day.

If you do the math, this amazing globe given to us to thrive upon for our short years is less than 8,000 miles in diameter. The depth of the atmosphere is about twenty-three miles. As you can see, the little six inch Styrofoam™ ball I intended to use to represent Earth in our mobile made it extremely tough to represent the thickness of the livable space around it. The math said that with a six inch diameter ball, which represented the 8,000 miles in diameter of Earth, then the thickness of the atmosphere around our mobile needed to be paper thin—Bible paper thin!

This realization took my breath away as I pondered the idea of how small our space really is. Taking this thought a bit further, I found it fascinating that God did not need to build a visible layer of protection to separate the livable space from space itself. We cannot see the dividing line with our eyes. Why is there just a limited amount of space for us to live? Why is not the entire universe made up of the same properties as the small area we refer to as the atmosphere? These were interesting questions indeed.

For now, let's take another look at the facts of our existence. There are currently about 6.6 billion people on earth. If you do the math, we could combine all of the people currently on the earth into a space that is about the size of ¼ square mile cube.

That means only one quarter of a mile east, west, north, and south, as well as one quarter of a mile tall.

With that understanding, and the size of the earth as previously discussed, does it seem possible for us to have a tremendous, or even measurable, impact on the earth's resources? My point here is not to rail in the face of the "green movement." In fact, I agree with it and drive efficiency on a daily basis, which is really what living green is all about. The idea is that we want to be more efficient on one hand, but also to simply create less of a load on the overall system on the other hand. One of my major talents is, in fact, building processes that ultimately cause more efficient lives and systems. Therefore, I am a big fan of green initiatives. What I don't agree with is marketing companies, governments, and organizations using tools such as this to manipulate us through fear to act in certain ways. Like I said, this is a whole different story, but the point is that we have been fooled, duped, and manipulated in our thinking. On our own, we have walked along ignorantly into the hands of those who stand to gain from our blank stares.

One example of this can be found in the concerns about the ozone layer around the earth. A few decades ago, it became big news that there were potentially dangerous holes in the ozone. The assumption was that we were chemically burning these holes with the excessive factories and use of toxins in our daily lives. The reality is that there were other factors that contributed to these findings. We had just developed the technology to be able to read the density of the ozone, and since there was no meaningful baseline to determine how much the layer had changed, the noted occurrences of thinning in the ozone were treated as a negative. Actually, what was happening was that the ozone layer was performing as it was designed to function by opening, shifting, and closing to allow gases to be released from the atmosphere. Just like our bodies are self healing, the atmosphere has also been designed to take care of itself. Nevertheless, just like we are seeing with the green movements, self-serving companies will jump on these reports to make the most of them financially.

If you are still in disbelief about the responsibility that companies and government have on our food supply, then read this quote from the CEO of a major fast food restaurant chain.

"Each item on our menu is engineered to produce a profit."

This quote is from a presentation given by the CEO of this restaurant chain at the International Franchise Association (IFA) Convention in San Diego, California on February 16, 2009.

Does that sound like a company that is first and foremost concerned about the health and well-being of its customers? This quote rang in my head. I wrote it down for you. The thing that is most astounding about this is that the majority of our culture would not question such a statement. Why? It is because we don't clearly see the connection between food and disease.

Interestingly enough, we think that is the worst of it when, in reality, the worst of it is the hundreds of thousands of people who are ailing and dying each year because they are unknowingly consuming animal flesh that has been inaccurately labeled as nutritional and necessary food. If you don't agree that restaurants have some ownership, along with all the other food manufactures and retailers, then I strongly disagree. I think any company that sells a product should take responsibility, along with unbiased steps to test and prove the validity and safety of their products. In other words, companies in the business of food should do the necessary research on their own to realize the contribution their products make in disease creation. They should also go to whatever length is necessary to prevent the harm of others through their business. Anything short of this course of action is unconscionable. Yes, these actions should be taken even if it means shutting down a company, or completely changing the course of a company's future.

When you combine these facts, it becomes obvious we do not have a resource problem; we have a thinking problem. Regardless of what you call it (ignorance, apathy, laziness, selfishness, bad habits, etc.), we have a big problem that has contributed to the entitlement culture that we current live in within our western society. Friends of mine have heard me call our land "zombieland." As a culture, we seem more interested in getting than serving, dreaming than doing, and consuming rather than assuming the responsibilities that have been bestowed upon us.

I want to wrap up this section with some definitions of a couple of terms that you will come across as you dig more and learn more about self healing. There is likely going to be a number of new terms that you run into. The ones below are essential to understand because of the implications they have on how our cultural perspectives have changed in terms of how we view health, medicine, and approaches to healing.

Allopathic is a term originally intended to point out how traditional doctors used methods that had nothing to do with the symptoms created by the disease, which meant these methods were harmful to the patients. Early on, it was quite negative in nature, and only in the last few generations has it become acceptable by the mainstream. Generally allopathic medicine refers to the broad category of medical practices that is sometimes called western medicine or modern medicine. The term allopathic has varying degrees of acceptance by medical professionals still today. I tend to use the term allopathic when I am talking about doctors that treat using pharmaceuticals (drugs or chemicals).

Non-allopathic would then be the opposite of allopathic. Non-allopathic medicines are also known as naturopathic, complementary, homeopathic or alternative medicines. Non-allopathic approaches have a much longer history than allopathic, and have only recently been displaced as the primary solutions to health-related concerns. Non-allopathic approaches have regained some ground with strong recognition in recent years, however, because they are less hazardous to our health. They actually provide some very promising results. These approaches include, but are not limited to, diet, herbs, metals, minerals, precious stones, essential oils, and non-drug-related therapies.

CHAPTER SEVENTEEN

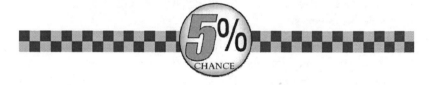

Twisted Truth

Listen closely the next time you hear a commercial for a drug. I heard one the other day, and the ad said, "Tell your doctor about <insert drug name>..." Why do we need to tell him about this new drug? Because he doesn't know anything about it and the whole perspective of allopathic medicine is symptom=drug. Thus, they are simply masking the symptom and not treating the source.

Furthermore, do you know that doctors are restricted on what they can actually recommend for your situation based on something called standard protocol, and if they recommend something outside of this then they could be putting themselves at risk of a lawsuit or losing their license to practice? Therefore, even though many doctors have learned many of the same truths that I have, they are restricted on how much of it they can share without jeopardizing their own sustenance.

Interestingly enough, I see a point in the future when the well-intended doctors could lose big time to the big pharmaceutical companies. When you think about it, we really don't need doctors in allopathy any longer. If you want to truly strip this down to what it is, simply prescribing drugs to treat symptoms, then why do we need doctors? What does the doctor generally ask you when he walks into the room? Doesn't he ask you, "What is wrong?" And are you not describing or self-diagnosing yourself by very nature of your description to the doctor? So what is to stop big pharmaceutical company from lobbying for legislation that will enable them to sell their drugs directly to the consumers, via a web portal, that would enable the consumer to simply type in their symptom and have a computer tell them which drug would be best for them? It may sound far-fetched, but I would be surprised if I am the only one thinking that would be a really profitable little web site.

We live in a culture that is so challenging on a day-to-day basis that we yearn for our next vacation to escape our normal existence. We no longer work for our own sustenance. Many years ago, people lived on a farm and were part of a bigger community. Within the context of this community, they would gain access to all of their needs. Primarily, however, they would supply themselves with food, water, and the basics.

Today, we tend to be segmented into what we are good at, what we do, and how we make money. If we were forced to provide for all of our needs on our own, it would be impossible for most of us. I am not saying there is anything wrong with making money in various ways, and then paying someone else to do things like tilling your crops and cleaning your clothes. I am simply making the point that we live differently today then we once did.

We get up in the morning and use any number of devices throughout our day that were designed to free up our time, and to make life easier and more efficient so that we have more time. Seriously, what is it that we are working so hard to free up time for? And when is it that we actually do the thing or things that we need so desperately to create time for? If you had more time, you might write a book, read a book (or thirty), spend time with family and friends in real relationship, serve the needy, start a business, do something great for your community or country, or maybe go on a mission trip down the block or around the globe.

I suppose the answer may be different for each of us, but I would contest that there is something more important happening as we go about our daily lives. Something that can happen in us regardless of what it is that we are actually doing. I say this because I have toiled for years attempting to earn the time to do the things I considered important. This became real to me on a trip to the ocean with my family one weekend. In this example, you will see my nature, and this is likely going to differ from yours, but hopefully you see the overall message that there is more happening in our midst than simply what we get to do. On this trip, one of the boxes we had planned to check on our weekend to the beach was to fly a kite. Our little kids had never been in an environment where this could be done easily. This was the weekend and we had bought a couple of kites to make it happen. The problem was that one of the kites broke quickly, and the other required a much better engineer than I to get it up and keep it in the air. It was like trying to control a remote control airplane that is headed straight towards you! Which way do I turn? What do I do? Many crashes later, I began to wonder why this wasn't fun.

This may seem incredibly unrelated, but it really isn't. In short, what I found was that my vision was to check boxes, not to enjoy time with my family and just be. For me, I needed to work on just being with my family and purposefully living out the joy God has enabled for us each day. I still have a box-checking propensity, but realizing my joy did not need to be tied to accomplishments or duties was a relief. I can go and have fun and crash kites with my kids and still feel like we had a great time just hanging out.

Living a healthy life can take some of your time. It can even take more time than eating unhealthy, but it does not have to. The first fast food appeared in the Garden of Eden. Seriously, Adam and Eve would take walks for their meals, right? Of course they did, and along the way they would simply pluck, pick, or dig up whatever they wanted to eat at that moment. Today, it is even easier than that. We just need to walk to the kitchen, open the refrigerator door, and pick what we want. I know we actually spend more time with our food because we like to combine things to make exquisite and wonderful dishes, but the extent of what we do is our choice. My point is that if you feel like you don't have time for this, then I would challenge what your time is for, in general. What is more important than whatever you can do with loved ones over a meal? What if your meals take an average of thirty minutes more per day than they currently do, would that really ruin your life?

We are surrounded by companies that are designing, manufacturing, and selling us stuff with the specific intent to make what should be questionable habits more efficient. We live for comfort. We will go to great lengths to protect our comfort, and that includes buying everything under the sun that we may or may not need to sustain our desire for more comfort. We protect our comfort. We worship our comfort. We even have comfort foods.

We don't actually use all the time we gain from our devices to do anything meaningful, though. In fact, we continue to buy more and more of these devices for the sake of having the latest toy. It is a status symbol. I personally think people that don't have cars are deprived. I can't imagine giving up that much freedom. But why do I think that way? Because I am programmed, thanks to our culture, to think that way. The people who choose to go without a car, an electric shaver, a ceiling fan, a microwave, or a television are not crazy. If you talk to them, they also do not feel like they are deprived. Surprise! They are getting it. They are beginning to realize their life is not about the next gadget or toy, or this or that. It isn't even about being comfortable or fully efficient. It is much greater than these.

You won't get there unless you begin to think for yourself about everything. You don't get there until you begin to question everything you are told, and the reasons for these things. And you won't get there until you put into question everything you think is real or truth. However, if you do grasp this, then you will immediately realize that you can eat whatever you want, or not. You can be whatever shape you want, or not. You can suffer and die of disease, or not. You can have a muscular stomach, or not. You can be vibrant and full of bounce and life, or not. It really is that easy. It is just a matter of saying "no" to our culture and the pervasive marketing messages, and "yes" to new thinking and a new perspective on what you do and who you are.

Do you still think I am off my rocker? Here are a few things we are confused about because of messages by someone. Most likely that someone is making a profit on the fact that people believe the wrong thing instead of what is actually true.

When we push from the terminal in an airplane, we are told to turn off and stow our electronic devices. We are led to believe that these devices mess with the controls of the airplane. That is not true. Everyone involved in designing airplanes either laugh or are offended every time they hear this because they know it is not true. One of the real reasons they require the devices to be turned off is because of the person-to-person rudeness of sitting in such close proximity to someone on the plane talking on a phone. Imagine a plane full of people talking on their mobile phones. That just won't work. It would be like the guy who thinks he is on the holodeck in Star Trek just because he has his iPod earphones plugged into his ears. Imagine a plane full of businesspeople and young punks all with active cell phones on a plane. How about the complaints the flight attendants would get because the phone coverage stinks, or someone is talking to loud? The other known problem has to do with the way the phones communicate with the cell phone towers and systems on the ground. Supposedly there is a question about how this may work. My guess is that the airlines simply don't want to deal with the effects and passenger confrontation, complaints, and just plain rudeness if it was allowed. After all, we have all been in a retail setting where the cashier was on a cell phone while helping us, or interrupted in a conversation while a friend sends a text message.

When we make a mistake and worship our food, comfort, possessions, dreams, or habits, we are bowing to false idols because we are idolizing something above God. That is the very basis of sin—worshiping a created thing over the Creator. When we do this, we feel the weight of our need for repentance and reconciliation to our true God. Interestingly enough, this weightiness seems to come from our guilt and shame. But, does it really? What we are crushed by is God's love. We are brought down by the fact that He loves us so much that even in the midst of our depravity, we are still fully loved.

It is more satisfying to eat less than it is to eat more. Seriously, I have done this many times. When you lay in bed with just a slight bit of hunger, you feel best and sleep best. It is a misconception that a full belly is most satisfying. In fact, in the long run it is quite the opposite. Even the short term results are not all that enjoyable.

In fact, we have misconceptions about many things in the world around us. We're fed an enormous amount of information that, in truth, is nothing more than the attempt to manipulate our way of thinking. For instance:

…the price of an automobile doesn't actually have a lot to do with the real cost of the design and construction of the car. The actual cost is driven more by the amount the market will bear. In other words, how much the target audience is willing to pay for such a car is going to have a bigger impact on the retail cost than the amount that is spent on actually building the car. All of this is known prior to even designing the car. If they can't get the math to work out then they won't allow the project to proceed.

…milk is not good for you and it is not a good source of calcium. In fact, due to the acidic results of consuming milk, the body loses bone density.

…schools do not need more money to improve their educational performance. A big budget will bring lots of amenities and unique opportunities for the students but creative, loving energy by the instructors and a passion for learning by the students does yield must better results.

…women tend to be consistent, predictable, and relatively easy to understand as compared to their counterpart. Men are general inconsistent, unclear, and seemingly devoid of overall mission and focus. We are duped into thinking that women are difficult to track with and understand when, in reality, it is the men that are struggling to even understand their own motivations, drives, desires, and feelings. I know from experience that I have reacted in a certain way in a given situation and then, even as it is happening, been questioning my own motives. A book called *For Women Only* by Shaunti Feldhahn is a great read. Nikki was so impacted by it that she bought a case and gave them to her friends.

...separation of church and state was actually created well after the founding of the U.S. republic. Many people believe that the founding fathers of America created the idea of the separation of church and state. The truth is quite the contrary if you do a little reading. Most of the original thirteen colonies required government officials to sign and oath of trust in Jesus Christ prior to taking office.

...children beyond preschool age do not actually learn at a faster pace than adults. It seems like it when they are young because they have so much to learn to catch up with the commonly expected set of knowledge and abilities. Once they catch up with the curve, however, the learning growth tends to slow down. This is not because the capacity to learn and understand has decreased, but rather because we spend less time investing in education the older we get. Thus, we learn less and at a slower rate. A good example would be for someone that desires to learn a foreign language. They could spend months or years with a few minutes a week or they could simply travel to the appropriate geographical location and spend a month there.

Hopefully I have astounded you with at least some of the fallacies we choose to believe, or that we have been forced to believe simply due to our own ignorance and the investment of others to make sure we think a certain way. What I want you to see is that we have certain beliefs about our diet and lifestyle that act as blind spots in our thinking. Some people or companies have paid big money to lodge these assumptions into our brains. We have the full ability and right to learn the truth and to take a different path with our lives.

I want to close by repeating my challenge from above. Do you want to be healthy? Do you want to enjoy a great body and be physically fit? Do you want to experience mental freedom like you have never had before? What is stopping you? I contest that it is nothing more than the realization that you can do whatever you want to do. Today, you can choose to ignore what you have learned about food, and begin anew with a lifestyle that will enable freedom and joy! As you do this, watch each day for the things that are not as you always thought. Take more joy in the fact that you are learning and growing as a person. This world is a clever dichotomy. We think it is all about us, our stuff, our food, and our time when, in reality, there exists a whole creative and wonderful canvas that is God's. Although it is in and of our lives, we tend to separate the two and focus more on our little stamp in time and space.

CHAPTER EIGHTEEN

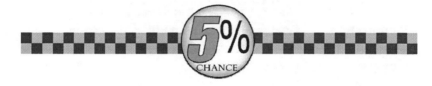

Life On The Go

I am often asked for advice on how to be successful in making healthy choices while living a busy, on-the-go life. One of the first things that I think about is the purpose of food and making sure this is correct in our minds first.

My family doesn't get together to eat. We get together to be together, and we eat as a method of relating and enjoying time together. We don't eat first for the satisfaction of the taste or texture of the food or the pleasure that comes from it, but we eat to fuel our physical body so we can achieve the greater endeavors our life has been purposed for. Our purpose is not food or eating. We design and reserve space in our home for food preparation and consumption. This space, although it is designed around the food, is not first and foremost purposed for supporting eating. It is purposed for creating environment. Think about a picnic table. It is designed to be sat around so that we face each other, have space for our food, and are able to focus on each other as we look across the table. If relationships were not pinnacle, then our eating environments could simply use a classroom or theater type of seating. Some of these seating arrangements are seen in some fast food establishments, but is likely designed for people who are forced to consume a meal alone. I suppose my question would be, why go to all the effort to have a meal if you can't enjoy it with someone? Is not food specifically designed to force our reliance on something external to ourselves, as well as to create a hesitation multiple times in our day where we naturally seek to be with each other?

I talked to many people looking for more options that support on-the-go living. Truckers are a good example, but they are no different other than they have a hyper need for more on-the-go flexibility. Truckers have it especially tough because their common stops and venues are filled with unhealthy eating options, and they also spend the majority of their time sitting. Consequently most truckers are out of shape, overweight, and generally in ill health.

I suggest truckers read to each other while they are driving. If they are alone, then there are a myriad of audio options that will enable them to continue their education. There are a number of great books that can be consumed while traveling. It may sound odd to mention this first, but continuing the education is a key component to them not giving up and just submitting to what they feel is impossible in their situation.

I then suggest that it is just as easy to stop at a grocery store as it is a gas station or truck stop. They have large parking lots and always have produce readily available. They need to really look at more food that is in its raw, whole state. For example, they could eat cucumbers like a carrot and red peppers like an apple. This is really the best way overall, but they will want to try to get as much organic as possible because it contains fewer toxins and tastes better.

Depending upon where they are (in terms of driving), they can also have stuff either sent to them or ready for them. If they stop at home regularly, but don't stay there long, they will want to develop a home on the road within their truck.

They need to get past the idea that BarleyMax® is too messy by simply developing a process for pouring and mixing it. This is really important, and if they get the right containers, it is very doable. Even if they only mix it when they stop, and mix a ½ gallon to sip on throughout the day, that would work.

Because the truck is moving most of the time, I think just making the leap to eating whole raw food is going to be the best advice possible. Nuts and dried fruit is good, but can very easily become too high of a percentage of the overall intake. They are also likely not eating the nuts raw and likely don't realize that most "roasted nuts" are actually deep fried and are therefore very unhealthy.

Burritos and various healthier packaged foods are fine as transitional food for a year or two, but ultimately they need to move away from these items. They also need to be really careful about MSG and other excitotoxins because these are very commonly in packaged and processed foods.

The biggest message all of us can take away from this is that eating "simply" is normally the very best for us and works in any situation. What I mean by eating simply is simply eating food the way it is picked off the vine, tree, or bush. A quick look, a wipe, and digestion begins! We can't get much simpler than this, and when we are living on-the-go, this is the easiest answer. The struggle is that mentally we need to make the leap to accepting the fact that a few pieces of produce can make up a meal. Once this happens, a whole new world of creativity opens up and we begin to realize the vast array of options that we have right in front of us.

I know this will be helpful as you travel about living this great life while choosing to see food as a tool rather than a reward, destination or purpose. Enjoy!

CHAPTER NINETEEN

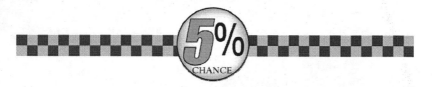

Simple Next Steps!

You have brains in your head. You have feet in your shoes. You can steer yourself in any direction you choose. You're on your own. And you know what you know. You are the guy who'll decide where to go.
-Dr. Seuss in *Oh, the Places You'll Go!*

As you begin this journey, let me be the first to encourage you to try to maintain focus on the things that you can and should do. If you get caught thinking about all that you are "giving up" or "can't do," you will quickly feel the sides of life folding in on you as if you are stuck, alone on a one lane road that leads to the most uninteresting, boring life you could imagine. Trust me, I can promise you from experience that although there are ups and downs along the way, I am so glad I took this path. I am more satisfied and full of life then I could ever have imagined.

I remember early on that I would literally starve myself. All I could think about were the things I normally ate, and I knew I was not supposed to eat those things any longer. The problem was that I didn't know what to eat! I mean, I knew I could have any produce I wanted, but that can seem so uninteresting when you are making the transition. Enter transitional foods!

I ate a lot of foods along the path that were good but not great. These foods served as good transitional foods. These enabled me to get to where I am today without feeling like I had to immediately remove from my diet all the foods that I ate the first thirty years of my life. One example is making a huge burrito with all the fixings, other than meat, and enjoying it. There is value in the produce on the burrito, but it is mainly rice and beans and those are fairly neutral. This is not a lot of nutrition, but certainly progress in the right direction. There is more nutritional value than a toxic load, however. Okay, great. I could do that. All I had to do was simply take the big hitters (toxins) out of my food and march forward. Remember, however, that transitional foods, by the very nature of the name, should be transitional—meaning, they are temporary.

With that understanding, here are the steps I would recommend you consider as you make the transition from what is likely a fairly typical western diet to something that may seem odd at first, but with retraining you will begin to experience firsthand the vital benefits.

Although I am presenting these steps generally in chronological order, some of them may require repeated attention as you progress.

If you read the Biblical book of James, you can see it is all about "doing." I love doing, so James is one of my favorite books. Too many of us skip that part where the Bible says "without deeds, ye have not faith." What we are being told is that if action does not naturally come from our faith, then it is not faith at all. Remember that if you are to be successful in this, the motivation must come from above. The last chapter in James reveals a process for being healed. It is clearly a two step process. Read James and notice the verse 5:14. God says to go to the Christian leaders and ask for them to pray. So, I suggest you begin your diet change with prayer and bathe your life in healthy prayer. God designed it as a mechanism of encouragement for us. Second, we must act in faith. Pray and then act. Do what you feel God is leading you to do. He will make it clear and He will show you the path to truth. If we are to find long term success, we must use the above verses as our motivation and confirmation. In this, we will act within the will of God and we will be successful!

Step 1:

Increase your intake of fresh, raw, organic produce. Make this as high of a percentage of your overall intake as possible to still be comfortable with your daily living. Commit to an emphasis on greens and try not to go a day without BarleyMax®. Begin experimenting with juicing and find some combinations you enjoy. Cut out all animal products in this step, which is anything that has a face or came from something that had a face. This includes dairy, poultry, and all other animal products. If you choose to include some transitional meat at this step, then consider one of the following seafood: salmon, flounder, sole, tilapia, or trout (according to the FDA, Office of Seafood, May 2001, these have the least amount of mercury).

Step 2:

Become a label detective. It is not necessary, but it is very likely that you will continue to eat some packaged foods. After ten years, I eat very little packaged foods. However, some great snack bars, and even BarleyMax®, are packaged foods. These examples just happen to have clean labels (good ingredients). The major consideration at this point is avoiding all excitotoxins. You will also want to avoid refined sugars and other obviously harmful ingredients. A good rule of thumb to work towards is that if you don't understand all the ingredients, then don't buy it. I commonly look ingredients up on the Internet if I don't understand them. You will learn a lot about various oils as you do this research and experience how you feel when you consume certain ingredients and oils. Be sure to pay close attention to how your body responds to whatever you eat. After a couple of times of not feeling well after eating something, you will often have plenty of motivation to simply choose something else.

Step 3:

Continue to Learn. This book covers the basics but it does not include your personal experience. Use this resource; mark it up and tag it as your personal handbook. In college, courses that are at the 100 level are generally as basic as this handbook is. The basis of step three is to continue the education while including your personal experience. Read at least two of the recommended books per year and begin to educate yourself, your family, and those around you as they have interest. If you don't have a community to lean on, then this is your opportunity to build one! Gather a group that expresses interest and help them. Every day we are faced with images, marketing, advertising, examples, opportunities, avenues, and habits that try to draw us down an unhealthy path. If we do not take a stand for what we know is right and true, then we stand a good chance of being courted back to the same, or similar, unhealthy lifestyle that got us to the point of asking for help. We have hosted a weekly food preparation evening in our home for many years. It is an open night, and it is encouraging for us as we help and lead others. It is important that you really put down some roots in this stage. Remember the Stockdale Paradox? We must maintain a stoic belief that we will prevail in this.

Get Ready!

Don't discount the need for physical changes that may need to take place in your home, kitchen, office, workplace, or other locations. Be creative and have fun. Don't feel like you need to purchase every piece of equipment right now. The most important piece of new equipment in our home has been the VitaMix®. We use it daily, and sometimes multiple times a day. There are other helpful things like good knives, a good juicer, and a food processor, but the VitaMix® takes the cake for the most used for sure. *Raw Food, Real World* by Matthew Kenney & Sarma Melngailis has a great list of equipment and food items to stock. It is not only a great recipe book, but a wonderful resource as well. Get a copy. Use it!

You may also begin stocking things like BarleyMax® at work with some mixing tools. You may also stock or take whole food snacks (produce) with you, or maybe stash some health snack bars or something. This sort of stuff will really help you as you transition. Sometimes we trick ourselves by not doing simple things like this and then use it as a continual excuse to not do what we know is the best for us.

Closing thoughts

Accept the fact that this is not just about the way you look or feel physically. This is as much a spiritual, emotional, and mental battle as it is a physical one. I can promise you my life has improved by leaps and bounds because of my clarity of mind and loss of fatigue. I think better, I feel better, and I relate in a more healthy way. Every aspect of my life is so much better! I know I am a better daddy because I can really think through my relationship with my kids when I talk to them in good times and in the face of challenges. I believe our lifestyle choices impact our access to God. When our minds are clear, we can seek and know Him in a way that simply is not possible in the cloud our culture would have us live within.

CHAPTER TWENTY

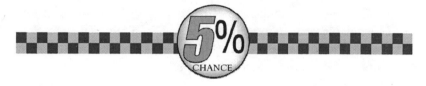

Frequently Asked Questions

1. **What are the real problems with animal protein?**

   It is my belief that the consumption of animal products is the chief toxin that we are regularly exposed to. I also believe, based on my research and the personal results that I've achieved, that the consumption of animal-sourced products causes over 90% of all diseases in the western culture. That is a big statement. We know that 98% of all medical care focuses primarily on disease-related care. I am suggesting that if we removed animal products from our diet and replaced it with a primarily plant-based diet that is free of chemicals or genetic engineering, we could nearly eliminate disease.

   Elsewhere I have given brief explanations about the problems and risks associated with animal proteins. There's not enough room or time in this book to delve any further into it. I want to ask that you read *The China Study* by Dr. T. Colin

Campbell. See the section on recommendations for specific info about this book.

2. **What are some good sources of protein?**

Dark, leafy greens are an excellent source of protein. The darker the greens the better. Spinach, broccoli, kale, peas and collard are all excellent sources of protein. Although greens have the most protein per calorie, some beans, lentils and potatoes are a good source of protein as well. The bigger question here is the determination of how much protein we actually need. I will address that briefly in the next question.

3. **How much protein are we suppose to eat?**

We have three beautiful children who have never had animal protein, and they don't even gorge themselves on the whole foods they eat. Therefore, there must be a sufficient volume of available protein in the produce we regularly consume. See the recommendations section for information on how to get some of our families favorite recipes.

Dr. Fuhrman answers this very question in *Eat To Live*. I have provided a summary of his answer below.

The recommended daily allowance (RDA) for protein has bounced radically over the years and the metrics for protein needs have changed from animal measurements to actual human measures which are assumed to be better or more accurate.

The World Health Organization (WHO) recommends only 5 percent of calories from protein. Even this estimate seems high to some experts. Most forms of produce contain at least 10 percent calories from protein which green vegetables average around 50 percent.

Dr. Fuhrman recommends a high-nutrient, plant based diet which result in the intake of about 40-70 grams of protein daily. He goes on to address the question of increased need for protein due to pregnancy or of an athlete. People in these situations need a higher intake of more than just protein so an increase in overall caloric intake (more good, healthy, whole, plant based food) is required. Within a healthy regime, the additional protein will also be delivered in adequate amounts.

4. **What are some good sources of calcium?**

Dark, leafy greens are an excellent source of calcium. The bigger question here is the determination of how much calcium we actually need.

According to the recommended daily allowance guidelines (RDA), a child should consume about 200mg/day of calcium. The recommendation scale increases by age up to 1200mg/day for adults over 50. It is interesting that babies who are attempting to grow an entire new body need so much less calcium than a full grown adult that is simply maintaining an already built body. This assumption indicates that calcium is only used for building bones which, of course, is false. The answer actually has more to do with our acid-forming diet than the specific growth needs of our body. A consumer of the standard western diet needs more calcium to overcome an acidic (low pH) environment in their body. In other words, westerners tend to consume a diet that causes or leaves an acidic environment in their body which creates the need for more calcium. Calcium is a tool used by the body to neutralize acid or bring acid to a high, more alkaline state. Therefore, when we eat foods that leave an acid ash such a meat, dairy, and sugar, our body pulls calcium from our bones to perform this necessary work. All of this leads to depletion of the bone density or less calcium in the bones.

The big marketing lie is on the billboards where the celebrities are marked with the white mustache. They are advertising how good milk is for the body, and by using celebrity endorsement to sell the idea, they're appealing to peoples' basic inclination to look up to, and follow, those they happen to admire. They do this knowing that when animal milk is consumed, we will need to deal with the resulting acid. They add a form of calcium to the milk, such as calcium carbonate, which can only be absorbed with sufficient resources of Vitamin D. The best source of

Vitamin D is through regular sun exposure, but of course we are told we should avoid sun exposure or lather up in sun screen, so we are generally deficient in Vitamin D as well.

On one hand the government is recommending, and even subsidizing, the meat, dairy, and egg industry so they can bring their harmful products to market at a competitive price. On the other hand, they are increasing the RDA for calcium to overcome the ill effects of these substances.

Here are some samples of good sources of calcium within a plant-based diet: seaweeds such as kelp, wakame, and hijiki; nuts and seeds such as almonds and sesame; beans; oranges; figs; quinoa; amaranth; collard greens; okra; rutabaga; broccoli; dandelion leaves; and kale.

Additionally, Dr. Fuhrman provides this chart in *Eat To Live* showing calcium content in 100 calories of various food items:

Bok choy 1055	Soybeans 134
Turnip greens 921	Cucumber 108
Collard greens 559	Cauliflower 88
Kale 455	Carrots 63
Romaine lettuce 257	Fish 38
Tofu 236	Eggs 32
Milk 194	T-bone steak 5
Broccoli 182	Pork chop 2
Sesame seeds 170	

The following research by others from Wikipedia further support my studies on calcium:

- Research has found an association between diets high in animal protein and increased urinary calcium loss from the bones.

- A diet high in fruit, vegetables, and cereals was demonstrated to result in greater femoral bone mineral density in older men, in comparison to a range of other diets.

- Diets high in candy were found to result in lower bone density in both men and women.

Mama was right. Eat your greens!

5. **Which juicers are better than others and why?**

First let me explain that a blender is not a juicer. Juicing is a method of separating the liquid from the fiber in living foods. There are no nutrients in the fiber. The fiber does have redeeming factors for sure, such as stimulating movement in the bowels by irritating them, but the juice is the live blood. Blenders simply pulverize the fiber and the juice resulting in a fiber-filled, pulpy juice. There is a lot of value in blending foods because it makes the nutrients more available for absorption when they are consumed. Blending and juicing also strips the nutrients of their protective shells, so they should be consumed as quickly as possible. If they are stored, then they should be protected as much as possible from oxygen and light. A good method would be to store juice in a dark container that is filled literally to the top before being capped off. This eliminates nearly all of the oxygen which can be harmful to the nutrients.

There are generally two types of juicers available. Most industrial (designed for high volume) and low-cost juicers use a centrifugal sort of mechanism where they cut the produce into tiny pieces and then spin these pieces rapidly, thus forcing the juice from the fiber. Most low-cost juicers use the centrifugal force methodology.

The premium type of juicers is a gear-driven type juicer. A gear-driven juicer is designed to grind the produce using a slow turning gear or gears which act against each other or the gear compartment. The key to these juicers is the powerful motor which enables the gears to turn slowly without bogging down or stopping. This eliminates nearly all the opportunity for heat to be generated while the produce is processed into separate juice and fiber.

There are generally three different designs to choice from, but only two of them are really realistic. The most expensive

(~$2500) is called a Norwalk. It is unrealistic because of the cost and the difficulty to use and maintain. The first juicer we had was a Norwalk that was loaned to us. They are wonderful juicers in terms of the quality of juice they produce, but they are super challenging to use and clean. The method of use is a two step process. The first step is inserting the produce into a shoot leading to a single slow turning gear-driven mechanism that grinds the produce into tiny bits. These bits are then gathered into a small canvas bag. This bag is then folded and placed into the second stage of the machine which is a mechanical press. The press squeezes the fresh juice out of the tiny bits from inside the bag. The porous bag material allows the juice to flow out onto a tray and eventually into a catch basin.

We have a funny story about the first time we used the Norwalk in our kitchen. I will just say that we had carrot juice and pulp all over the kitchen, on the cabinet doors, ceiling, countertop, floors, in our hair — everywhere!

The two reasonably priced and realistic gear-driven juicers are known as the Champion and the Green Star®, which is also called the Green Power®. The Champion has been around for the longest, and was one of the pioneer machines in terms of bringing gear-driven technology to the marketplace. It is a single gear machine, so the produce is pushed down the throat of the machine and is mashed by a single gear. The turning action of the gear forces the mix toward the end of the machine. The juice is allowed to drain through a screen while the fiber is pushed towards the end of the machine where it exits into a catch bowl. Overall the Champion is a good machine and can be purchased new for under $300.

The ideal juicer on the market today is the Green Star® juicer. The Green Star® is very similar to the Champion. However, it uses a twin gear design where the produce is crushed in between two slowly spinning gears. The mix is forced down the machine and a screen allows the juice to drop while the pulp continues along and out the end. The twin gear method increases the juice yield and continues the low temperature, low speed methods that are common for the gear-driven machines. A Green Star® juicer can be purchased new for under $600.

One of the big benefits of a gear-driven juicer is the ability to make nut butter and fresh fruit sorbets. Some gear-driven juicers will also allow juicing of fine greens, such as wheat grass. Although none that I know of are really good at juicing greens, there are some that have optional attachments that allow for juicing of greens. We use ours for frozen fruit sorbets regularly. When fruit begins getting over ripe, we prepare it for freezing. For example, we peel bananas and put them in bags for the freezer. Strawberries are cleaned and topped before bagging and freezing. We then pull the mix we choose from the freezer and create a sorbet (using our gear-driven juicer) or smoothie (using our Vitamix®).

Centrifugal-type juicers tend to induce a bit of heat into the produce because they are spinning so rapidly. This heat does have an impact on the quality and life expectancy of the resulting juice. Most information that I have read suggest that there is about a 20% - 30% loss in overall quality. Clearly the juice from a centrifugal type juicer is still very good quality and beneficial, especially if it is consumed soon after the juice is extracted. Centrifugal juicers made for home use usually cost significantly less than a gear-driven type juicer. Centrifugal juicers are typically $90 - $140.

My recommendation is to purchase a gear-driven juicer if you can afford it without a strain. If you want to start with a centrifugal-type juicer, then that will be fine, but plan for a 6-12 month life with regular use. During that time you can use my next tip to find a gear-driven juicer for less cost than retail.

Search on-line at auction sites such as eBay.com or Craigslist.org to see if you can find deals on gear-driven juicers. Stop at local garage sales or thrift stores occasionally also. Success in this would be to find a good functioning used Champion for around $100, or a Green Power® for under $200.

Since I discussed blenders in this answer, let me also recommend that you put a Vitamix® on your "to-buy" list. A good blender, such as the Vitamix®, a good juicer and a quality set of knives will be your kitchen staples as you learn to live and eat healthfully!

6. **Are there certain foods that I should be aware of combining for positive or negative results?**

I don't believe it is nearly as important as some people may think to avoid certain food combinations. I am not saying that I don't think this is a valid subject. What I am saying is that it simply does not fall on the priority level anywhere near the things that someone new to this lifestyle should be considering. As you gain knowledge, this may be one of the electives that you pick up and study but, like everything as it relates to your diet, let your laboratory of one (yourself) be part of the equation in determine what works for you and what does not.

When I was diagnosed, I was encouraged by Hallelujah Acres to limit high-sugar foods, even raw, whole food sources such as carrot juice. To be honest, I scoffed at this. My response was something like this. "Look, if I am going to give up all this other stuff and eat what feels like a limited spectrum of foods (a mind-myth that I thankfully busted through), I am not going to concern myself with what I eat or when I eat it."

I am not advocating that this was a wise or justifiable attitude. Clearly it may not have been in my best interest. I could have followed the recommendations of the experts more closely for sure. Maybe I did, yet I just wanted a bit of control in the situation.

I think a good point to realize here is that it is easy for us to eat all fruit. Fruit is sweet and is designed to be a treat. Therefore it should only be a small fraction of the total diet.

So, to get past my less-than-optimal attitude on this subject, there are some things to learn in this area. I just don't feel like it is a starting point for someone trying to get into living a healthier lifestyle. The last thing I want for you is to finish preparing a wonderful meal, and then suddenly realize that you are eating two things that may be more difficult to digest or assimilate.

7. **Have you ever considered having someone from the medical community partner with you to formally document your story?**

   It seems like so many people could be helped if it was fully validated, and since you have all the medical records, this should be possible.

   We actually got to shoot a TV show with a big northwest news station a few years ago. It was a neat experience, but we were surprised that much of the show spoke of people that were failing in the methods that were considered state-of-the-art. At the same time, very little emphasis was put on the fact that we had beat melanoma and had not used the conventional medical protocol. To me, it just felt like someone needed to step back and look at the big picture of what was being shown and make some reasonable assumptions.

   In terms of documenting it with a reputable medical source, I would be interested in this, but sadly, I am not sure who or what conventional medical organization would align with me. The problem for their marketing departments (yes, these are companies – medical companies with marketing budgets) is that they would not be able to draw a line to any dollars by promoting my story. Success stories are always great, but they would want the bottom line to point more people to use their modalities. In general, other than monitoring and maybe cases of partnership where people combine conventional treatments with prevention, I don't know that they would be able to make the leap.

   There may be some non-allopathic organizations that would jump at the chance, and I would enjoy those opportunities, but I am not sure that this would lead to increased validation or credibility of my story as I am assuming the person that asked the question is getting at.

8. **What are your thoughts on the various methods for detoxifying?**

Our bodies are in a constant state of detoxification. We live among toxins so we have to constantly deal with this. Thankfully, we have a lot of mechanisms built into our bodies to do this work.

I know the question is more in terms of focused or intentional detoxification. I am not a big fan of detoxification diets or periods because the implication is that we are choosing to do something radical on a temporary basis to overcome long term problems. I have heard people say that they detox one month a year, or one week a quarter, for example.

Detoxification takes months and, in some cases, years. We can choose to drop the coffee or sugar habit and only deal with the outward signs of detox for a couple of days, but the reality is that it takes weeks or months to clean our system of all of these toxins.

Our fat cells store toxins, as well, so when we make positive changes in our diet and lifestyle our bodies respond as if it is spring time! We begin to clean house. The body opens up those fat cells and begins processing the toxins that we have stored there. Sometimes this process will result in us feeling worse at certain periods because we are working through the process of removing these toxins from our system.

I am a big fan of a long-term detox approach. What that looks like is really very simple. It is a matter of providing more nutrition to our bodies on a daily basis than the toxic load we are exposed too. In other words, if we are experiencing a load of say 14 toxic buckets per day, then we would want to make sure that we counterbalance that with more than 14 buckets of nutrients. Clearly the actual measurement of these is dependant upon the severity of the toxin, or the strength of the nutrition in consideration, but you get the point.

There are a couple of approaches. We can increase the amount of healthy stuff we are doing or eating, or, we can reduce the toxic load on our body where we have control over that load. The majority of the toxic load comes through the food we eat. Most of the rest comes through the air we breathe.

I have heard stories of sever detoxification. Roger Recovers From Aids is one of my favorite stories about detox, but I believe there is a less uncomfortable way of achieving the same result.

Some clinics encourage extended water fasting as a method of detox. This can be very uncomfortable and dangerous. Furthermore, it only addresses half of the problem. Water fasting eliminates most of the toxic intake, but it does not improve the nutritional side of the equation. When you look at it in these terms, you can see that fasting from toxic food and beverages is great if, at the same time, it is combined with intake of highly nutritional foods.

If the detoxification symptoms become greater than a person is comfortable with, then they can simply slow the process by eating more cooked foods. Like everything I have written, I think the focus should be on long-term success rather than short-term, fit-into- my-bathing-suit results.

9. **How long should it take for food to go through my body?**

Technically, this is called "frequency." It is the transit time from the point of entry to the point of exit (defecation). It is a fairly common thought but rarely asked — by men at least!

Here is the deal. Your digestive system is a tool to provide your body with nourishment. Many people see it as an extraction tool, and it does work as that, but that isn't the primary intent. What I mean is that we see it as a machine to extract the nutrition from the things that we eat. Case in point: you eat a hamburger and think that your body will pull the nutrients from the lettuce, tomato, and ketchup, and of course the ever important protein from the meat (hopefully you know that is a myth by now), and then send it into your blood stream and throughout your body for whatever all those various organs and internal mechanisms need such things for.

Unfortunately, that is the way most of us use the digestive system. It is actually designed to quickly capture the nutrients, which are chiefly mechanically extracted with our teeth in our mouth. There is some minor chemical breakdown that happens in our stomach, but not nearly as much as we commonly burden our stomach with. In other words, the right foods provide nutrients that fit exactly with our bodies. The stomach and the rest of the system doesn't need to take a lot of action to extract the nutrition.

I will use myself as an example since my body has been a living laboratory for over nine years…well, nearly forty if you count all the years I was eating like the billboards told me to.

I head to the bathroom every time I eat. It is a natural reaction for your body to clean out the old and make space for the new. The actual transit time (time it takes to pass through) should be well less than 24 hours. Any guess what the typical transit time is for a westerner's diet? From what I've read, it is about seventy-two hours. Here is something else to think about. What happens to a bunch of fresh raw produce if you put it in the blender, and then let it sit out at room temperature for twenty-four hours? Not much right? In fact, it will most definitely still contain some life. Now think about the burger. If you blend that up (you will naturally have to add some soda pop so it will blend properly in the blender, right?) and set it out on the counter at room temperature for three or four days, what is it going to look and smell like?

The problem is that certain foods make your digestive system sluggish and it does not push as aggressively as it normally would. This is caused primarily with low-fiber foods. Did you know that animal products do not contain a bit of fiber? Fiber is what activates the contractions within your intestines. It keeps things moving on through. Produce is all fiber, other than the water which is packed with the essential nutrients.

The nutrient-packed water is the life blood of the plant and our bodies. The fiber is just the carrier so wouldn't it make sense that it would cause your intestine to contract and push it through?

The intestine is designed to be a one-way tool. Once the food passes a certain point, toxins and additional water should be added to the intestines, but nothing should be coming the other direction. Everything should be on a one-way train to the light at the end of the tunnel. What happens when food lingers in the digestive track is that it builds up a high level of toxins, and these toxins are then able to work their way back into our system.

So, how do you increase the trips to the outhouse? Eat more fiber! It will stimulate your intestines and encourage the movement of much of the muck and pus that builds up from tons of carbohydrates and animal protein. Talk about an easy way to drop a few pounds quickly. Just increase your intake of raw, plant-based foods. There are also some herbs that can help stimulate the bowels into action. Hallelujah Acres has an herbal fiber blend that works really well. If you persist in eating a western diet then you may consider a periodic cleanse with something like this. I am not saying it is good to eat like our culture does, but the idea of all those toxins building up inside is nasty, not to mention very unhealthy.

Since we are in this region, some of you may know of or wondered about rectal itching. It is caused by parasites (more toxins) escaping (being forced out) during the natural detox process. It isn't supposed to last long, but can be expected if you make some improvements in your eating habits as your body begins to clean house.

10. **What does the term "organic" really mean, and who polices the use of this?**

Organic, to me, means that food is grown based on the original intent. For example, a seed is put in the ground, watered, and allowed sunlight until it produces a result such as fruit. Within the understanding of being organically grown, this process must be free of fertilizer, other chemicals, or additives in the soil or during the growing process.

I will get back to my definition in a moment, but for now, let's look at the perspective of other sources. The diversity of opinions or applications of definitions is interesting, maybe even a bit scary. This information may cause you to question the use of the term "organic" all together. Hopefully, in the end, these facts will force us to realize that everything comes down to the basis for truth that each of us uses. If that basis varies, then the results will vary equally. Where there is no apparent basis for truth, we find people who make decisions based on self-serving factors. These people live completely devoid of the natural conscious responsibility that a person who understands foundational truth demonstrates.

Dictionary.com has several definitions for "organic." Definition number nine states: "Developing in a manner analogous to the natural growth and evolution characteristic of living organisms; arising as a natural outgrowth."

This is a fancy way of saying what I said. I agree with this definition.

Definition number eleven from dictionary .com says, "Pertaining to, involving, or grown with fertilizers or pesticides of animal or vegetable origin, as distinguished from manufactured chemicals."

Basically, what it says is that we can and should call something organic provided whatever we use as fertilizers or pesticides comes from a plant or an animal. This is not shocking on the front, but the implications are tremendous. Basically, what it says is that it is okay to label something organic provide the ingredients used to accelerate growth are from so-called natural (plants and animal) sources. What bothers me is that we could so easily include animal substances in this mix. Little do most of us know that one of the most-used substances from an animal for fertilizing is excrement. Looking just at the economics, this is a very reasonable way of getting growth encouragers such as nitrogen, phosphorus and potassium into the soil. There are a number of negative effects of this, but without belaboring this any longer, I just want to make the point that we can actually grow great produce without using animal products for fertilizing or as a pesticide.

From Wikipedia under the heading "Organic Food":

Organic foods are made according to certain production standards. For the vast majority of human history, agriculture can be described as organic; only during the 20th century was a large supply of new synthetic chemicals introduced to the food supply. This more recent style of production is referred to as 'conventional,' though organic production has been the convention for a much greater period of time. Under organic production, the use of conventional non-organic pesticides, insecticides, and herbicides is greatly restricted and saved as a last resort. However, contrary to popular belief, certain non-organic fertilizers are still used. If livestock are involved, they must be reared without the routine use of antibiotics and without the use of growth hormones, and generally fed a healthy diet. In most countries, organic produce may not be genetically modified. It has been suggested that the application of nanotechnology to food and agriculture is a further technology that needs to be excluded from certified organic food. The Soil Association (UK) has been the first organic certifier to implement a nano-exclusion.

The inclusion of this from Wikipedia leaves more questions than it provides answers on, but I felt that including it here would help lay the foundation for how really vague the definition of organic really is. Furthermore, I wanted to show how daunting it would be to manage the implementation of the standard related to growing something organic. The main point that I would like to expand upon is the idea that organic is something new. The Wikipedia text makes is clear that organic is much more common and historical than the new conventional methods of chemically affecting the crops and soil.

I will close my definition phase here with another quote from Wikepedia. I think this is interesting because it shows the five general guidelines or requirements for becoming organically certified.

From Wikipedia under the heading "Organic Certification":

Organic certification is a certification process for producers of organic food and other organic agricultural products. In general, any business directly involved in food production can be certified, including seed suppliers, farmers, food processors, retailers and restaurants. Requirements vary from country to country, and generally involve a set of production standards for growing, storage, processing, packaging and shipping that include:

- *avoidance of most synthetic chemical inputs (e.g. fertilizer, pesticides, antibiotics, food additives, etc), genetically modified organisms, irradiation, and the use of sewage sludge;*

- *use of farmland that has been free from chemicals for a number of years (often, three or more);*

- *keeping detailed written production and sales records (audit trail);*

- *maintaining strict physical separation of organic products from non-certified products;*

- *undergoing periodic on-site inspections.*

In some countries, certification is overseen by the government, and commercial use of the term organic is legally restricted. Certified organic producers are also subject to the same agricultural, food safety and other government regulations that apply to non-certified producers.

In my definition above, I describe a perfect world sort of scenario. We put a seed in the ground, the rain waters it, the sun shines upon it and after a certain amount of time we harvest fruit. Knowing that God made us, that He made food for us, and that He designed a way for us to be able to exist and enjoy that food with little to no effort on our own, should increase your worship of Him. I know it does for me!

One of the big things we need to understand as we look at organic farming or agriculture is what I call "factory farming." Not too many years ago, most produce was grown on small family-like farms. It was more of a garden-like environment. Farms found that growing certain crops in and around and even mixed in with others helped the yield, as well as provided protection from bugs. They also learned that picking the produce at a certain time of the day resulted in less bugs being captured within the produce. Ultimately, these families may have gone on a walk for most of their meals, quite literally eating as they worked. Regular, sit-down meal preparation may have been an occasion rather than common place.

Fast forward to today, with miles of land skimmed flat and tilled, turned, planted, watered and harvested by machines. Of course in this factory farm, we need a mechanism to protect the crops. The corn and peas really enjoyed growing together on the family farm, and they provided necessary protections, but within thousands of acres of corn there are no peas in sight. So we need to introduce some chemicals to protect the corn from the bugs. While we are at it, why not also include some additional chemicals that will help the plants grow more rapidly? After all, if I can turn the crop more quickly (similar to manufacturing turns in a factory), then I can yield a better result for the shareholders (it is all about money).

I lightly covered the part of the question having to do with regulation of the established standards. Given the length of my answer already, I will limit my response here and just encourage you to read up on the role the United States Department of Agriculture (USDA) plays in managing the organic standards within the U.S. and the International Federation of Organic Agriculture Movements (IFOAM) for international information.

11. **What can I do to repair a chronic kidney problem?**

See my answer to Question 13 below. I have a friend that had a chronic kidney problem, which he was told was incurable by his doctors. He started juicing and eating greens, and over an 18-month period he lost about 200 pounds and cured his kidney problem as well as a long list of other ailments. Question everything. Just because someone says something is impossible doesn't mean that it actually is really, truly impossible. It likely means that either they don't know the way, or they don't have the energy to make it happen.

12. What can I do if I have had a surgery that has removed an organ such as my thyroid?

This is a great question. I don't have any in-depth answers because I think I would get into the zone of prescribing if I did. My intention is to educate and illuminate, not to prescribe or direct. If we get a part of our body chopped off, cut out, or removed then, in many cases, the rest of the body has mechanisms to be able to overcome these situations. Certainly if someone has their heart or brain removed, then that would pose a rather difficult dilemma, but other, less critical organs or parts, can be overcome.

What is most important in these situations, and in the point of any diagnosis, is that we do not lose hope. The greatest hope that I know is in choosing to live as healthy as possible, given the choices that we have at our fingertips, and to avoid as much toxicity as possible. Beyond that, we do not have any control. However, because we do not have ultimate control, does that give us license to ignore what we can do? I think not. I encourage everyone, in every circumstance, to do all they can and leave the rest to our Maker. At times, it is going to feel like we do a lot of the work, and at other times we are going to realize that we do very little of what needs to be done. Also, at times, we are going to experience loss due to someone being unable to win their race against disease or illness.

It is in times like this that we can question the sovereignty of God. After all, I just said that we have to do all we can and leave the rest to Him. Please don't fall into this trap. He is fully sufficient.

I know someone who came to some of our classes that had a very serious cancer diagnosis. He looked in very tough shape from the day that I first met him, and I doubted his ability to win his fight. Nevertheless, I knew there was no better path than to do what he could, considering his circumstances. He eventually lost the battle, but he did so peacefully and without a tremendous amount of pain. I don't know if the cancer had just spread too far or if the modalities of the medical treatment he was also enduring were the cause. I also do not know the extent to which he really adopted what I did.

His family could have cursed God for not filling the gap completely so that he could continue in life. The problem with that thinking is that it is very selfish. What they would be saying is that they want God to come and be a part of their life and their story. They would be saying that they are the center and the one of most pre-eminence. Instead, we should be honored to know that we get to be a small part of God's big epic story. We should see His grand canvas stretching beyond the space of time and realize that upon that great canvas is our little scene. We can take great honor that we get to be a tiny part of His grand plan. When we do lose our life, or a loved one loses theirs, we should continue to rejoice in our God because He has created all, delivered us, and loves us. Nothing remains unfinished that matters. Jesus' last words were, "It is finished."

13. Are there certain veggies that help overcome disease?

All of them! Let me share with you my perspective on the problems with our health care system as it does actually relate to this question. One of the main problems is that we call health care, well, health care. It isn't health care at all. Dr. Tel Oren recently said in a seminar that 98% of the energy expelled within the hospitals and clinics of the western world is done combating disease. Should we not call this "disease care" instead? After all, we are working on attempting to fix disease, right? Where does disease come from? Disease comes directly through, and from, the lifestyle choices that we make each and every day as we walk through our lives.

If you want cancer, then a recipe is readily available for you. If you would like heart disease, diabetes, or multiple sclerosis, then step right up and pick up a recipe. We know how to create each of these. Why then is it so difficult to reverse-engineer our actions to the point where we accept and understand that we are quite literally creating these diseases within our own bodies? The problem with that is everyone would be forced to accept the fact that nearly all physical health conditions are a result of their own actions. That is like saying a dirty word in church. Don't tell people what they are doing wrong or they might feel bad. That would just be politically incorrect.

Instead, let's tell the people that they need more doctors and pills so they can feel well again. Let's burden the entrepreneurs and their companies with the responsibility of balancing an impossible budget by demanding health insurance that is laden with high costs as a direct result of poor lifestyle choices.

We need to take a systematic approach to health care. It needs to begin with the understanding that there are three separate elements to the care. The first is disease. The second is accident, and the third is prevention.

These are the three pillars that our health care system should be built upon. Accident care represents less than 2% of the overall expenditure of the system. Thankfully, we have great hospitals, doctors, and drugs to help us through times of serious trauma. Yes, I did just say that! Remember, I am a racecar driver. I enjoy the comfort of knowing that emergency rooms today have the capabilities to deal with such things. I don't want any of that to change. I just want us to look at it differently.

Prevention needs to take center stage. It is going to happen first and foremost through good education, like what Hallelujah Acres and other organizations are teaching. This is teaching that emphasizes the power that we have in our choices about our food and our lifestyles. This will lead to a revolution of sorts where we will force the suppliers of our food to give us what is healthy, in addition to what they can make a profit on, instead of just the latter.

This sort of approach will also prevent the bloated bureaucracy of Washington D.C. from forcing businesses to pay for disease care they simply can't afford. If that does happen, then it would be the undoing of the entire entrepreneurial system that built this country, because there would no longer be any motivation to build or grow. Why? Because the precedence would be such that the government would simply take anything that we earned. Furthermore, the people would feel the backlash of such a decision because they would quickly learn that the small businesses they work for cannot afford the disease care coverage the government is requiring, and will either respond by lowering wages or closing the doors. Either way, the people lose. We need to step back and institute long-term sustainable results and quit working for momentary gain.

So, what would I eat if I had a disease? Well, I do have a disease. I have lots of them. One is cancer, and what I do for that is I eat lots of raw, fresh, organic produce. Is there certain produce that brings about better results? Yes! The best, most nutrient-dense foods on the planet are dark, leafy greens of all sorts and kinds. I eat them and enjoy them in abundance. Second to that, I am not sure the mix of food I eat has a big impact. I primarily eat what looks, smells, and tastes good, provided it is in a whole food state.

14. **I have heard you say that drugs don't cure. If they don't, then what do they do. And how do I achieve healing or cure?**

There is no drug on the planet that cured anything, nor has there ever been to my knowledge. That may be difficult to get your arms around considering how much we are taught to trust in those colorful pills, but it is true. The effect of drugs is simply to change the symptoms that we experience.

Isn't it interesting that we see an ad for a drug, and it is happy and positive, and then we turn the page only to see a fine printed page full of all the side effects? What are these side effects? Well, they are actually the primary effect of the drug. In among these primary effects is a masking of your symptoms if you are one of the unlucky ones.

Does that sound backwards? It should, but it is not. The unlucky get their symptoms masked by a drug so they keep taking the drug forever. If they were cured, would they not stop taking the drug and go on about their lives? That is why they are unlucky because they stop looking for the cure.

If they got to the end of their rope, with no possible drug in site to cure them, then maybe, just maybe they would attempt some alternative methods such as changing the way they eat. This is again another interesting use of words. Why do we call anything other than conventional medical treatments that have only been around for a few decades, alternative methods? We do that because we are copying the marketers, and that is the way they speak, so we just copy them. The reality is that many of the natural methods, especially dietary and lifestyle choices, are much more common and have more history than any of the conventional treatments.

The only way we can achieve healing or a cure is through the work of our own individual body. Our self-healing mechanisms need to do the work required to achieve healing on a daily basis. If those mechanisms are compromised or weak, then they are going to slowly lose the battle. The best we can do is to strengthen our self-healing systems so that we maintain a healthy physical state at all times.

15. **What were the first indications that you were successful with your diet changes?**

Within a few days, I felt much better than I had in years. I began sleeping better almost instantly, and I felt some of the mind fog lift in just a few days. My skin tightened, I had hope, and I just felt good. I am still amazed at how resilient our physical bodies are. We can abuse them for decades, and then after only a few days of eating healthy, we can get some amazing results.

16. **What is the difference between consuming animal flesh and fish?**

Dr. Campbell, in *The China Study*, covers the problems with animal protein in good detail. He also presents the information in a way that is easily understood and motivational. Hallelujah Acres also warns strongly against the intake of any animal protein. The thinking from these, and many other professionals and individuals, is that the animal protein actually causes many of the physical problems that we experience. I have yet to read anyone that puts fish in the same category, however. The main concern with fish, as I understand it, is that many of the fish species contain a high amount of heavy metals that are toxic to our bodies. Mercury is specifically discussed because it is found in many different types of sea life.

17. **Explain GMO.**

According to Wikipedia, a genetically modified organism (GMO), or genetically engineered organism (GEO), is an organism whose genetic material has been altered using genetic engineering techniques. These techniques, generally known as recombinant DNA technology, use DNA molecules from different sources, which are combined into one molecule to create a new set of genes. This DNA is then transferred into an organism, giving it modified or novel genes.

For example, this technology has been used to create a "terminator gene" within certain crops. Corn is one that has experienced heavy genetic engineering. The terminator gene was designed to create infertile crops. In other words, the seeds would yield one cycle, but if the farmer attempted to plant the terminator-infected seeds, they would not grow. Why would anyone do this? The reason is that the companies can put a patent on the seed (or at least attempt to), and thus take ownership of a particular crop seed or version of the seed. In doing so, they force the growers to return year after year to buy their seeds.

As if this technology wasn't bad enough, you may have noticed that I talk about this in the past tense. The reason is that the terminator gene presented some serious social problems if it somehow spread or infested other non-GMO seeds—which, of course, it did. So, how did they respond? They designed another type of impotent seed. This one will grow normally and will reproduce in subsequent years, but only if the farmer purchases the proper fertilizer. This magic mix comes, of course, from the same company trying to dominate the seed market in the first place. Now, they don't actually have to manage the seed stock any longer. The farmers will do it for them, and return year after year to purchase the magic mix to make the seeds grow.

You vote in the way you spend your money. I urge you to demand non-GMO products in all your purchases. The implications of GMO are limitless and discomforting.

18. **What is wrong with soy products?**

The biggest problem with soy products is they are nearly all GMO. Tofu, a common soy product, represents only part of the greater bean or edamame (soy). Tofu is made by coagulating the juice from soy beans. This is done using various different methods, but is questionable secondarily to the fact that it initially came from a GMO source, because it is no longer a whole food and requires significant processing to produce.

There are lots of options to every soy product, and therefore I see no reason to take any risk by regular consumption of soy or soy products.

19. **Can you explain water quality? It seems like there are so many options and I am confused.**

I have been asked by a bunch of people to represent or endorse their water machines the last couple of years. The main push is in the area of water ionizer machines. These machines are fascinating. They can literally change the state of plain water and make a highly alkaline water that has some benefits to our bodies (because those eating the standard western diet tend to be acidic), or turn the same water into an acid strong enough to sterilize.

The problem with the ionic machines is that they don't perform the same function as a distillation process, which is to remove the toxins. Distilling is not perfect either, because it also removes the necessary minerals that exist in the water. Drinking only distilled water for long-term can actually leech our bodies' resources rather than fill them. If you are using distilled water, the latest recommendation includes adding some sort of liquid mineral back to the water after distilling, such as WaterMax® by Hallelujah Acres.

With the best technology that we have today, it seems that the following process (in this order) would yield the most ideal water, other than water directly from a plant:

- Distillation
- Ionization
- Add living minerals back

The problem is that the equipment for achieving the above is not readily available. It could be easily built, but it just has not been done yet.

Remember that the absolute ultimate best water on the planet for our consumption is found inside living produce. Something magical happens during the photosynthesis process. The result is a living water found only within a living plant. That is where the nutritional value comes from with our consumption of produce. The produce is made up of fiber and water. The fiber is simply a carrier for the nutrients, and the nutrition is found in the water. Don't be fooled into believing that you need a certain amount of plain drinking water everyday. The more raw, whole foods you eat, the less necessary supplementing with drinking water is.

20. **Why is it that many vegetarians are just as unhealthy as others? That fact deters me from even trying a vegan or vegetarian diet.**

You may come across "social vegans" at some point. Nikki and I visited a vegan pub recently for fun. My guess is that the proprietors created the establishment mainly out of concern for animals. I mention this here because social vegans tend to be rather unhealthy. The reason is because they focus mainly on protecting the animals rather than consuming a healthy diet. In other words, they don't generally see anything wrong with eating animals from a health perspective. The result is a diet that is laden in processed foods and empty calories. They remove the toxins, but they don't load the system with highly nutritional foods that are low in calories.

The other reason that we see vegetarians in a sad physical state is chiefly due to the fact that most vegetarians continue to eat dairy products. Dairy contains a concentration of animal protein and is therefore just as harmful, if not more so, than an actual steak.

21. **What role does spiritual health play in healing?**

I don't feel that it is possible to live completely counter-culture without the help and support of God. For that reason, I think that a spiritual awakening or journey is necessary for each of us as we endeavor to live a more healthy life. Even still, we can easily get wooed into marginalizing the long term, systemic, life-changing message about the relationship between our lifestyle choices and our health state. Just like any other aspect of our lives, we must rely on and trust in the Creator, not creation or created things.

CHAPTER TWENTY-ONE

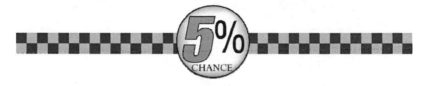

Recommended Learning Tools

Today we're blessed to have a wealth of information available to us, literally at our fingertips. I am of the opinion that you don't have to necessarily agree with, advocate or endorse everything in a book to glean some knowledge from it. The books I recommend are those that I found to be the most truthful. However, even books that don't appear on this list can have nuggets of useful information.

For example, I read *Brain Rules* by John Medina and learned a lot from it. Nevertheless, it was sort of like visiting the National Natural History Museum in Washington, DC, where they call all sorts of animals "family" with the clear and bold intent to teach us through conjecture that man came from animals by evolution. The first chapter of *Brain Rules* covered the effect of exercise on the function of the brain. It is the most comprehensive explanation on the relationship between exercise and brain function I have ever read. Even the author, however, stated that the text, and even all the science combined today, only scratches the surface. He said that at best we should assume what we know is only a very small, nearly immeasurable bit, and that we tend to look at facts and knowledge singularly instead of dynamically amongst the others axioms acting in a particular situation.

While I found *Brain Rules* interesting, I could not help but be a bit distracted and question the foundation of all the information simply due to the pervasive evolutionary theological bent. My point here is that I was able to read the book, and learn from it, even though I knew going in that it was foundationally flawed. It is nearly impossible to read anything that does not contain at least a bit of untruth, even if it is not intended to be so by the author, publisher, or editors. The obvious exception is the Bible. It, by its very nature, is infallible.

Before you dive into the list and make plans for what you will do next, I want to warn you of one other thing that has the ability to hinder us in our path forward. In fact, this little thing can cause us to slip, falter, fall, or worse—to be infected by apathy.

Most of us idolize comfort. We desire to have things done for us, and we work momentarily in anticipation of the promised coming comfort. It could be a meal, a movie with the family, a vacation, or any number of other things. It is clear that we desire comfort over discomfort. When given the choice, the answer is not even a consideration. The reality is that growth always requires pain. There is nothing you have ever learned through education, experience, or revelation that was not delivered on some painful path.

2 Timothy 4:3 says, "For the time is coming when people will not endure sound teaching, but having itching ears they will accumulate for themselves teachers to suit their own passions, and will turn away from listening to the truth and wander off into myths."

What if I had asked the doctor that removed the mole from my back to have it checked for cancer if he could use something not as sharp, scary, or seemingly painful as the scalpel? What could I suggest that should be used instead? How about a magic wand? In part of my mind, I want to avoid all discomfort at all costs. In the logical part of my mind, I understand that I must endure some pain in order to progress.

My point here is that we can easily deceive ourselves by creating excuses in our minds for why this or that is okay. For example, I have been told many times by someone that they are following the "blood-type diet" so they can eat <fill in the blank>. Or another one is that this particular thing <again, fill in the blank> isn't really that harmful in their view, so they are going to keep doing this and just modify the basic foundational truths they read. Each of these is like a major blind spot in our minds. It prevents us from seeing the truth that is right in front of us. We press on while dragging carnage from our choices along with us when freedom is quite literally as simple as letting go of the false truths that we have been programmed with.

For this reasons, I provide a list of educational recommendations in this section. If you work through these teachings, then you will be armed with the knowledge to be able to determine truth and error in other educational opportunities you choose to participate in.

While I have arranged the books in this list in the order they should be read by people who are just beginning down this path, I would also suggest reading each of these regardless of your place, or the amount of time you have been attempting to live a healthy lifestyle. The one exception is Dr. Russell L. Blaylock's *Natural Strategies for Cancer Patients*. Although this is a great book and filled with great information, it is highly technical, and it is of the most use primarily for allopathic practitioners and people struggling with cancer.

I have also included a list of recipe books we use. This list is simply a sample of the hundred or so recipe books we have collected over the years.

All of these publications should be available at your local library. Or, if your budget and space allows, I recommend purchasing and keeping copies of these on hand for reference and review.

The China Study by T. Colin Campbell
If you like "the data" as much as I do, and you appreciate factual information collected from a reasonable sample size and presented in a simple format, you will enjoy The China Study. I have been told that the source of this data is the largest human study undertaken to prove the relationship between our diet and disease.

Eat to Live by Dr. Joel Fuhrman
What's wrong with the food pyramid, calorie counting, fats, and fish oils? What is this about the calorie-counting myth? Do we really need to eat that much? This book is one of my favorite references for my own education and for assisting others. For example, I love to reference the "Health = Nutrients / Calories" on page 7, or find out how much I should weigh on page 22, or the nutrient density chart on pages 120-121. Dr. Fuhrman has an active practice with thousands of patients, and within the hardback cover of this book he shares his findings from years of research, trial, and error.

The Hallelujah Diet by Rev. George Malkmus, Lit.D. with Peter & Stowe Shockey
This is a heartfelt, interesting, story-like publication that demonstrates the overall raw vegan health message. It is as good as any other publication I know of and uses facts, testimonies, stories, results, history, and a biblical foundation. Our story happens to be included in the cancer section of this publication (page 68). The inclusion of our story does not elevate this text on my list. This is a very comprehensive book which combines science, results, and strategies, and can serve as a great handbook for major change in your health. The Hallelujah Diet replaces a previously written and wonderful book titled God's Way to Ultimate Health. I would still strongly recommend this book because it is bigger and includes a lot of valuable information.

Excitotoxins by Dr. Russell L. Blaylock
Read what the food manufacturers are adding to the products to entice us to eat them often and in large quantities. Arm yourself with information that will enable you to make sense of at least some of the confusing food labeling. I am convinced that excitotoxins are directly related to the increase in diseases such as Alzheimer's and Lou Gehrig's disease among others.

Natural Strategies For Cancer Patients by Dr. Russell L. Blaylock
Dr. Blaylock talks through the synergistic potential of using natural approaches to fight cancer alongside the conventional medical treatments. Natural Strategies for Cancer Patients is an enjoyable read. It explains the impact and necessity of nutrition in the fight for success over cancer in a scientific (and extremely technical) way that no other book I have read does. Dr. Blaylock clearly wrote this text with the intention of assisting in bridging the gap between non-allopathic and allopathic approaches. Dr. Blaylock also wrote Excitotoxins, which is in my top five must-reads for anyone truly interested in improving their health.

Roger's Recovery from Aids by Bob Owen, Ph.D.
I have a special affection for this book because I am the type of person who often finds myself doing what others say is impossible. The book is a true story, and it is as much a love story between old friends as it is a story of the process two men took to prove that AIDS is a lifestyle disease and does not have to be either irreversible or a terminal ailment. I read this book in three hours. Once I started it, I simply could not put it down.

Fast Food Nation by Eric Schlosser
The title of this book is a bit deceiving, but it is nevertheless a worthwhile read. The thing it seemed to best identify for me was the industry momentum caused by our cultural choices. These have made it nearly impossible to eradicate sickness, and the ingredients in our diets that are responsible for the disease. Learn how our food industry is controlling our economy, legislation, and most discouraging of all, using up people (mainly migrant workers) as if they were mechanical machines that can be thrown away for a newer version.

Pregnancy, Children, and The Hallelujah Diet by **Olin Idol, N.D., C.N.C**

Dr. Olin Idol does a wonderful job of dispelling many myths in this book. He reviews the basics of such things as natural birthing options, breastfeeding, toxicity, supplements, and more. He also includes instructions on how to transition your child from breast milk to solid foods, and at what age and period of development to consider changes of these sorts. We especially appreciate this work because we talk to so many families who say their children simply won't eat a healthy diet. We know, through experience, that children will not starve themselves by refusing to eat healthy food when no unhealthy options are available. The reality is that the parents simply won't lay down the law for their children, chiefly due to their misled training when they were raised.

Raw Knowledge: Enhance the Powers of Your Mind, Body and Soul by **Paul Nison**

Paul interviews a variety of people who have implemented a primarily, or all, raw food diet. Paul is a Hallelujah Acres Health Minister, and travels full time, speaking and teaching about living a healthy lifestyle. He is also a big fan of Ann Wigmore. She and Dr. William Howard Hay were well ahead of their time with their work and teaching a century ago in the area of raw, whole, living foods, and the advantages of eating this way for nourishing the human body.

Living Food Cures: The Amazing Stories of 11 People Who Beat Disease Using Raw & Whole Foods by **Joseph R. Farinaccio**

This is an interesting read and contains stories from several people I know. You will be motivated and inspired by these stories. I encourage you to contact these people and bless them if their stories helped you. Most of them have contact information in the book.

Good to Great: Why Some Companies Make the Leap...and Others Don't by **Jim Collins**

This book recommendation may seem a mistake at first glance. After all, Good to Great is a business book, and Jim Collins' work has all been in business-related efforts. What you will find when you read this book is a list of foundational life truths. Sure, they apply to business, but they first apply to life. I address one of these, called the Stockdale Paradox, in this book. If you want your life to go from good to great, you first need to learn the basic elements of a good life versus a great life.

Why Christians Get Sick by Rev. George Malkmus, Lit.D.

Rev. Malkmus addresses what should be one of the topics Christians consider in their work—to eliminate all false idols. He talks about the basic biblical reasons for a diet and lifestyle free of the consumption of animal products. Rev. Malkmus also reviews the basic approach to living a healthy lifestyle, and the justification for doing so as a believer in Jesus Christ.

Health Via Food by William Howard Hay, M.D.

Dr. Hay was at least eighty years ahead of his time. He wrote this book in only three weeks, back in the early 1900's, after spending over twenty years attempting to successfully apply the allopathic approach to medicine (symptom + drug = allopathic method). He then spent over twenty years applying natural, diet, and lifestyle-based remedies similar to what we know today with great success. Although he didn't know about the harm caused by animal protein, he was bold enough to face down the status quo and the ridicule of the allopathic practitioners who disagreed with his unconventional approach.

Terapia Gerson Cura Del Cancer Y Otras Enfermedades Cronicas by Alan Furmanski

Alan is a melanoma survivor and a health advocate primarily in Spanish-speaking cultures. He introduced himself to me through a mutual friend, and we built a relationship through the years as we both fought to beat the worst, fastest moving cancer. I am very proud of Alan and the work that he continues to do. Since I am not fluent in Spanish, I have not read this book, but Alan has told me that the foundation of it is in and around the teachings of the Gerson Institute which is very similar to Hallelujah Acres.

No More Bull!: The Mad Cowboy Targets America's Worst Enemy: Our Diet **by Howard F. Lyman with Glen Merzer and Joanna Samorow-Merzer**

Howard Lyman is famous for his comments on Oprah regarding the consumption of beef, which lead Oprah to say she would never eat another burger again (because of Mad Cow disease). These comments led to a lawsuit which they ended up winning, but it just shows how big and powerful the food industries are. Howard grew up on a ranch in Montana, and shares about his experiences in raising cattle and farming. It is interesting to learn about the transition from sustenance farming to production farming or ranching. The farms of today are huge food manufacturing facilities. The ground is the work surface; the seeds, rain, and chemicals are the additives; the grain or produce becomes the packaged product.

RECIPE BOOKS:

Below is a list of recipe books we selected from the hundred or so that we own. We generally categorize all of them by recipe difficulty and time to prepare. Many are simple, some fall in the middle, and only a few are really challenging. I have given you a mix of all in order of priority as used or liked in our home. Enjoy!

The favorite recipe book in our home!

Raw Food, Real World **by Matthew Kenney & Sarma Melngailis.**

We have really enjoyed every single recipe we have ventured into from this book. The raw lasagna (page 173) is probably my overall favorite raw food dish to date. The recipes in this book can be somewhat difficult to prepare. If I had to rate them on a difficulty scale of 1 to 5, they'd be a 3. However, they do a great job of laying out all the ingredients and the tools for the kitchen in this book. It's just a must-have piece for any healthy kitchen. Don't skip reading the opening pages.

We also enjoy using recipe books by Rhonda Malkmus and Julie Wandling, HM, which are available through Hallelujah Acres.

I really like Julie's books because they are full of really simple recipes that anyone can make. Julie is a mother of two growing boys, and her books are very personal. They tell about her story and are inspiring kitchens across the land. Look for the following titles, **Thank God for Raw**, **Healthy 4 Him**, and **Hallelujah Kids**.

Rhonda's primary book, **Recipes for Life** is wonderful. It reminds me a bit of the Betty Crocker cook books from when I was growing up in the kitchen with my mom. We've had great results and it's not too technical. Be sure to note the 5-star rating system used in this book, because it does a great job of helping to educate what foods and combinations are the best for our bodies. Try to lean on the 5-star recipes for staples and splurge with the recipes of lower stars occasionally. The Hallelujah Acres Colonial Bread is amazing. Rhonda also has a really great holiday recipe book that we have used many times. This book is titled **Hallelujah Holiday Recipe Book**.

Vice Cream by Jeff Rogers

Vice Cream should be on the recipe shelf of every vegan. It is packed full of seventy dairy-free frozen dessert recipes. About half of them are raw, but I can promise you all that I have tried are wonderful. Just because you are vegan and eating healthy doesn't mean you can't have ice cream. My favorite is the basic vanilla.

Living On Live Food by Alissa Cohen

This is another wonderful recipe book we have added to our library recently. We have made several of the recipes and enjoyed the results.

Raw: The UNcook Book: New Vegetarian Food For Life by Juliano with Erika Lenkert

I met Juliano in his San Monica restaurant, and from just a few minutes with him, he seemed like quite the character. Nevertheless, he makes great recipes which result in cuisine-like meals. Just be ready for some hours in the kitchen before you crack this one. The recipes are tough, daunting, and include many uncommon ingredients. If you do get it, try the juice called "blood"—it is wonderful.

Juicing For Life: A Guide to the Health Benefits of Fresh Fruit and Vegetable Juicing **by Cherie Calbom and Maureen Keane**

This is a really useful digest, not only for great juice recipes, but also for disease-related information. The recipes in this book are organized based on the ailment one is trying to address or improve.

How We All Went Raw: Raw Food Recipe Book **by Charles Nungesser and Stephen Malachi**

This is a really fun book with many simple recipes that result in some tantalizing meals.

FAVORITE RECIPES:

Visit this page for a bunch of our **favorite recipes**:

> **www.freggies.com**
> *(look for the link to the recipes)*

This is a wonderful resource because we have loaded many of our favorite recipes for sharing. It also saved a lot of space in the book, and you can get the latest updates like the ones I added yesterday that were not there when this book was published.

We are also considering doing some food show videos, too, so watch for that.

Here is an approach to a basic salad:
Of course, this isn't the only thing we eat, but getting hooked on good salads is one of the best things that will happen when you begin to make changes in your diet and lifestyle. I estimate that I have had about 5,000 salads over the past ten years, and never once have I eaten the same salad twice. Talk about variety!

Rule number one: enjoy it. If not, then change it!

We choose to always use 100% organic ingredients. The flavor spectrum on conventional produce is the chief reason why people salt their tomatoes and avocados. It is because they don't have any flavor! Eat organic!

Lettuce: Favorites - Butterleaf (nice, thick, and leathery). Sometimes, you might skip the lettuce and have a "no lettuce salad."

Tomatoes: Favorites - Heirloom by far, but cherry tomatoes are great, and there are others that are good, too).

Cucumbers: Remember, there are 170 different ways to slice, cut, chop, etc. Sometimes peel, sometimes not...

Onions: I enjoy green onions, but I prefer slices of red onion.

Carrots: We don't use these often in salad, but there are a ton of fun things you can do with them in terms of shape, etc.

Avocado: They need to be pretty firm or they are gross, but if they are right, they are amazing. You can also make a guacamole and top the salad with it and some salsa.

Spices: Sometimes I just go in and begin dumping various spices, but one that sticks in my mind is fennel seed. It is nice if it gets a chance to soak it in, for instance, some rice wine vinegar or some other liquid in the bottom of your salad. It really brings out the flavor.

Sauces/dressings: Go wild here, but remember that the more exotic you get with your sauce, the fewer ingredients you need to be really satisfying. You can kill the value of some ingredients by over-dressing. I love just freshly squeezed lemon, and depending upon the salad, no dressing at all can be nice.

Toppings: We have a cupboard full of nuts, seeds, raisins, flax, etc. I may take chopped walnuts with oranges on one salad, with cashews or sunflower seeds on another salad, or a combination of any of these. We also really enjoy a raw taco mix made mainly from walnuts. Topping your salad with it makes it a lot like a taco salad.

Shocking: For fun, try blending your salad sometime. You can easily get hooked on these...

ENJOY! And remember to visit www.freggies.com regularly to see our favorite recipes.

AUDIO/VIDEO RESOURCES:

God's Way To Ultimate Health by Hallelujah Acres, starring Rev. George Malkmus, is the video our family watched that blustery, but insightful, Christmas day of 1999. It is basically an overview of what the whole Hallelujah Diet® and Lifestyle message is about. It has been updated since and is even better now. The information is irrefutable and has universal application to all people. If you are starting down this path, I would suggest getting a copy for your library and schedule a couple hours to watch it about every three to six months during the first two years. I am still amazed how much I learn as I watch it the fifty-sixth, fifty-seventh, or fifty-eighth time.

The Miraculous Self-Healing Body by Hallelujah Acres includes professional insight from four medical doctors on the subject and relationship of diet and disease. These doctors are Dr. Neal Barnard, M.D.; Dr. John McDougall, M.D.; Dr. Joel Fuhrman, M.D.; and Dr. Russell Blaylock, M.D. This video is narrated by Rev. George Malkmus, Lit.D., and is obviously produced to support the Hallelujah way of teaching, but the truth in the message is nonetheless powerful and inspiring. I think our culture's respect for doctors is part of what makes this particular educational piece carry such impact.

Super-Size Me was released in 2005, and is a story of a guy that eats only McDonald's food for thirty days. The criteria included several things, but one was that he had to try everything on their menu during the thirty-day period. He only ate at McDonald's, and his entire experiment was documented along the way. It was really an interesting and worthwhile investment of a couple of hours. It helped me come up with my version of understanding in regards to food production in our culture today. It goes like this (in my mind at least): there are basically two rules that matter in food production in our culture. The first rule is that the food cannot cause immediate death to the customer. That's right, you may die from eating it over and over, but that seems to be okay in our society. It may be loaded with MSG, and you may feel terrible, but as long as your taste buds are tantalized during the courtship process of eating, the food will sell. After all, if there are side effects to the food we eat, there most certainly must be a pill we can take to curb the side effects (I won't go on about the profit machines called pharmaceutical companies and how a drug has never cured anything…). The second rule is that the food has to be profitable. These companies are in business. Food manufacturing is about money. This is not a healthy vs. non-healthy issue. Even the farms are making money! These are just the facts, and it is our responsibility to be aware of them. Food is a very big business and the results of the profit machines are not always healthy for us. (Available in DVD format from any public video rental location and may be found in some health food stores).

Food, Inc. was released in theaters June of 2009. It is the highest quality and most comprehensive movie I've seen showing the relationship between our buying choices and the habits of the food industry. It is argued that the food industry is leading the population astray with unhealthy, yet profitable, foods (what they call food), though they would defend themselves by saying they are simply producing the things people want to buy. Learn more at www.foodincmovie.com.

Fast Food Nation started as a book by Eric Schlosser, but was later made into a B- grade movie with a cameo by Bruce Willis, where he tags the famous American meal as the $*!# burger. I think the tag-line they have for the movie is great, "Would you like lies with that?" By the name, you would believe this film has a lot to do with fast food or fast food restaurants. In reality, it has more to do with the sad story of the mechanism or machine that quite literally uses up and eats humans in the process—namely and chiefly U.S. migrants from Mexico. If you can watch the last ten minutes of the movie, and still stomach lunch that includes some form of animal products, then you have scales of steel and calluses that need a grinder.

Eating by Mike Anderson is a very informative video that uncovers many facts the meat and dairy industries don't want you to know; things like the fact that the products of these industries are the biggest cause of disease and death in the western culture. Mike Anderson discusses the link between diet and disease in

America. He also opens up the hidden door behind which we find that our farms have turned into factories whose chief purpose is feeding the animals we eat.

Suggested Web Recommendations:

Hope4Health.org
You may have already visited, but this is our little web site.

Hacres.com
This is Hallelujah Acres main web site. There are tons of testimonies, resources, products, and BarleyMax®! Tell them that Jerrod and Nikki Sessler sent you if they call. Everyone in the call center knows us, and I always try to make time to go down and see them in their office area each time I visit Hallelujah Acres. They are a great team.

Fitday.com
This is a neat little on-line tool to track what you eat and learn nutritional information about your diet. One of the coaching things I recommend for people who are dealing with physical issues is to document what they eat or drink for three weeks. This is a great tool in determining where the gaps in nutrition may be, or where some areas of toxicity or excess may exist.

Soulbyte.com
I was recently introduced to this neat web site. It is a really neat way of learning scriptures relate to various circumstances we face. Quickly download audio files filled with encouraging scriptures related to the selected topic.

TheTruthAboutYourFood.com
Dr. T, the creator of Ecopolitan, a completely organic, vegan and raw food restaurant, spa, and shop in Minneapolis, Minnesota, is one of the most educated and rational scientists alive today. He questions all that seems obvious to the rest of us (which I think is good), and what he learns in doing so is astounding. The older I get, the more important I realize it is to question all of our assumptions. Why? Because most assumptions are driven by marketing dollars that intend for you to think a certain way, but their way may not be truth. Visit

www.thetruthaboutyourfood.com to learn more about Dr. T, and watch his teaching via video.

Good 2 Go Café

We have a vision to place healthy cafés across the country in strategic community locations. These cafés will be owned, manned, and staffed by people with a passion for teaching and assisting people in eating healthy food, as well as learning more about the food they eat and how the lifestyle they live impacts their overall health. Part of the café concept is that we will also deliver fresh, organic produce regionally in and around the café through Freggies. So, check out www.freggies.com and tell us if you are interested in starting a produce delivery service or launching a healthy café in your region.

Additional Web Recommendations:

One of the great things about writing a book is that you can put whatever you want in it just because you want to. Below are some great, though somewhat unrelated, web links that I thought would useful to share.

Freggies.com

This is an organic produce delivery services. Nikki and I started this company in an attempt to meet the needs of busy families who wanted access to great quality organics at a bit lower price than retail, and on their terms (pick what you want), with free delivery! We plan to expand delivery to many cities in the future. Please do me a favor and pronounce "Freggies" correctly. It sounds like "veggies." Just drop the "V" and add an "Fr" from "Fruit" or "Fresh". Fresh Fruit & Veggies = Freggies!

EmeraldCitySmoothie.com

I know the owners of this through the franchise world, and they are really great people. A friend from high school also owns some of the locations around my neighborhood. Smoothies make a wonderful meal. We own a couple of VitaMix® machines, and make lots of smoothies at home, but we still find time to go to ECS regularly. What we have found is that eating out is a social thing, so we really want to go places to be social more than just filling the tummy. It is great if we can go somewhere and grab something together and still have something healthy. This is a good example of just that.

HomeTask.com
This is a franchising company I started a few years ago. HomeTask is a portal that enables members to manage all the service of their homes, buildings and properties. We also offer franchise opportunities for various service brands through HomeTask so you, a friend, or a relative could apply to begin a franchise in your region.

eHow.com
This is a neat little site to learn just about anything you want. Check it out and enjoy. If you join and write some of your own how-to's, you can make money.

MarsHillChurch.org
My family attends Mars Hill church. All the teaching is posted on-line and amazing. If you have ever desired to know Jesus, understand redemption on a daily basis, walk with and really dig into a true relationship with God, then I would recommend you check out a Mars Hill campus or on-line. If a campus is not close to you, then grab a group of friends and set a time to gather weekly to watch the teaching and discuss it (this would be called Mars Hill Underground, and I have heard there are hundreds of groups like this worldwide). Reach out to your community and love them just as Jesus does us!

APPENDIX A

Jerrod Sessler Cancer Diagnosis Timeline:

This section is a reference for those who are really interested in the process we went through and the choices we made. You have to realize we didn't really know much about, nor believe in the idea of the natural self-healing ability of our bodies at the start of this. The education process weighed heavy on the front end of this process to get us to the point where we trusted what we thought to be true enough to place the balance of my life in the hands of that truth.

12/31/98   First doctor's visit when the mole on my back was discussed. I mentioned the mole on my back that was bothering me with an itching sensation. This doctor looked at it and said it looked fine. He did not document this, but did note discussing my dry skin.

For anyone interested in the resolution to this obvious failure by someone in the medical profession, I want to elaborate a bit here. In other words, did we sue the doctor? The answer is no. There are fundamentally two reasons. The first is that I struggle with the criteria our culture uses when engaging the legal system. I am not saying that there is not just cause for such actions at times, but I don't know if this was one of those. The second, and more resounding, reason is that I believe this was providential by God. Sort of like when he closed Pharaoh's mind to the common sense of letting the Israelite slaves go, even when God's wrath was upon him and his Egyptian people repeatedly. I believe God blocked the doctor from warning me about this mole, possibly along with everyone else, until it was the right time to illuminate the course of action I needed to take. The reason I believe this is primarily because I know myself, and I know I probably would not have taken such serious action had I not been faced with a literal death sentence. Had I thought maybe I had a 50% chance of making it, I would have taken it. Thus, I would now be dead because it would not have worked. We know from history that melanoma returns with a vengeance, and the patients are rarely spared when conventional medical treatments are enacted. Now, I get to live a wonderful life with a gorgeous wife, incredible children, and loving family. I get to glorify God (exclaim Him to others) and live out His joy for me daily.

10/12/99 I showed my mom (who happens to be a nurse), the mole and said it was itching. She stated she would get me into a dermatologist as soon as possible. I trusted her and agreed. My mom had seen the mole before, but it had been a long time before, and she had chiefly just seen me backing up to wall corners to scratch it.

My weight at this point: 217 (the highest ever….)

10/13/99 Mom went to work the next morning and promptly called to schedule an appointment with Dr. A. However she was booked more than a month out, so Mom asked who could get me in, and Dr. B had an opening on the 19th. Dr. B was a new doctor, so Mom couldn't ask anyone about her. However, Mom went by the clinic reputation of hiring good doctors, and she made the appointment, time being of the essence.

10/19/99   I saw Dr. B and she set up an appointment to excise the lesion. She stated that she didn't think it was anything, but it could be a basal cell carcinoma. I told her that my maternal grandfather had a history of melanoma.

10/24/99   I called Mom, wanting to video my excision. She didn't think Dr. B would appreciate that, but told me I could call and ask them.

11/4/99   Doctor's notes: Excision lesion/mole on back (1.5 x 4.0 cm) excision.

I called Mom from Dr. B's waiting area to come down and observe the excision, since we weren't recording it by video. They took me back while Nikki stayed in the waiting area, and Mom went back also. Dr. B came in and inked the shape and size of her intended incision. Dr. B's assistant numbed the area with a local anesthetic, and Dr. B came in, gowned and gloved. She made slow scalpel cuts to excise the mole, which came out in one piece. She also made small scraping and digging type cuts at the body edge of the cut in some areas. Dr. B sewed two layers, pulling my back together fairly firmly. Before the stitching was complete, I complained that I was starting to feel it, but I was fine and she was to continue. She and her assistant applied a pressure dressing, and told me to keep it on for at least twenty-four hours before removing or showering. During this visit, I stated that Mom was to have any reports or access to my records while we were in the room.

The five Clark levels of invasion for melanoma:

Level I: Melanomas confined to the outermost layer of the skin, the epidermis. Also called *melanoma in-situ*.

Level II: Penetration by melanomas into the second layer of the skin, the dermis.

Levels III-IV: Melanomas invade deeper through the dermis, but are still contained completely within the skin.

Level V: Penetration of melanoma into the fat of the skin beneath the dermis, penetration into the third layer of the skin, the subcutis.

11/6/99   I asked Mom if she could take out the stitches, and she said she wouldn't mind at all. I said it would save me a trip downtown. I also asked her to cancel my appointment, which she did the next morning.

11/11/99   *Doctors notes: Dermatopathology Report by Dr C – Malignant melanoma Clark's Stage IV - Read out as 1.14 mm in depth and within 1mm of the excisional margin.* (see note at the end of the chronology addressing level and stage issues / contradiction)

Mom called to see if the report was in yet, and when she was told that it had not come in, she asked to be called when the pathology report did arrive. The person at the other end of the phone said fine. They did not say that Dr. B was out of town, or that Mom could not have the report or that they needed a release.

11/16/99   Biopsy results visit with Dr B. After initially discounting the severity of the melanoma, Dr B consulted with Dr A and decided to send me to the Big Melanoma Clinic. She did a full body skin check for other lesions and reminded me to use sunscreen lotion. She also sent me for a chest x-ray and liver function tests for metastases.

I want to note here that I included the reference from the doctor about using sun screen as a point of clarity. I did have a few sunburns as a child and as I grew up. I grew up primarily in the Pacific Northwest where short bursts of sun, rather than regular baking, are common. I do not, however, believe that the skin cancer is a direct relationship to sun exposure. The cancer I had was caused by excessive toxins within my body during a time when I was nutritionally deficient and could not prevent the creation and spreading of the cancerous cells.

11/16/99   After not hearing for such a long time, Mom called to get the report results. They said that it had gone to Dr. C and gave her the number. She called and they faxed the report right over saying that it had been sent to Dr. B long ago. When she received the fax, she was shocked.

Mom called my sister to see if perhaps Deirdre knew if I had gotten any report. Deirdre called me as I was heading southbound on the viaduct's top level along the beautiful Seattle waterfront, and I said I had not heard a word. I knew that Mom had called her, and I could hear in her voice the news was not good, even though she didn't mention it directly. Then Mom called me and told me to call Dr. B's office and ask for the results. I called Mom back later and said that I was going to pick up Nikki, and would be seeing the doctor at 4:30. I asked her if she would come down.

When I arrived, I called Mom and she came down, meeting a worried Nikki in the hall near the office. We all went in the room together. Dr. B came in and told us the news very calmly as if it was no big deal. She said she would just do a wide excision in the office and that would be that. She measured the width she wanted to make, the wide excision pointing to an area approximately two centimeters from the original incision in all directions. Mom said nothing in this visit except to ask at what point it becomes surgical instead of dermatological. Dr. B answered that usually they (dermatologists) took care of it until it became a skin graft situation. She said she would have to do a full skin check today. At this point, Nikki and Mom started to leave, and I said that since Mom gave birth to me and Nikki sees me everyday, there was no reason for them to leave. Dr. B looked me over and found one other suspicious area on my left buttock that she thought would need to come out. She left the room for a few minutes and then came back and said that she had spoken with Dr. A, and would refer me to the Big Melanoma Clinic for possible lymph mapping. Dr. B seemed to take this quite lightly and stated that where she came from, they didn't consider this level to need lymph mapping, and insinuated it was overkill. She said her assistant would get the number for us. Mom volunteered her extension.

11/17/99   Mom knew someone with the number for the Big Melanoma Clinic, so both Nikki and Mom called. The assistant at the Big Melanoma Clinic was very nice, but said I couldn't get in until the 30th. Mom explained that this had been cooking for a while, and that we would be available any time if she could find a cancellation spot. The lady said if Mom could make copies of the records and fax them to her and hand-carry the slides, she could look for another spot. Mom got the chart, made copies and faxed them to her, and in the meantime she reworked her schedule and called us both back to say the new time and date would be 11/23/99 at 10:30.

11/18/99   Mom tried to reach someone at Dr. C's office, but got only voice mail, so she left a message saying she would like to pick up the slides about 12:00 noon. When she arrived at the doctor's office, they were unaware she had been coming because that nurse was off and the voice messages had not been listened to. They did look for them while she sat a bit. Soon they came out saying the slides went back to Dr. B's office as per her protocol. Dr. B's office had not said anything about the Big Melanoma Clinic needing records, or that they had the slides and would be glad to provide them to us.

11/19/99 Mom called and asked to be able to pick up the slides, and Dr. B herself spoke to Mom about the fact that she needed a written release. Mom asked if my statements in our visits were not enough. Dr. B said no. Mom asked if she had to call me off the job to come down and fill out the form. Dr. B said it could be faxed. Mom still had to reach me out on the road to have me go home to get the fax and return it signed, etc. This was the last straw for her. She started to cry and had difficulties the rest of the day. She took a walk at lunchtime and stopped back by Sandra's office in staffing to see if she could get the day off to go with us to the Big Melanoma Clinic. Sandra looked at her and asked what was wrong, and Mom just burst into tears. It seemed as if Dr. B and her office staff just didn't care, and were more worried about protocol than the patient or patient care or patient needs. To top it off, they turned Mom in for getting the chart and copying it for Dr. D at the Big Melanoma Clinic. First off, she did nothing until the pathology report was late and no one had called. She followed all the rules to the "T." The fact that there was no cooperation or concern left her feeling that if she requested anything, it would not get done.

A staff member in the human resources department called Mom down to speak to her about ordering a chart, and copying it when it was not her doctor's chart duty. She just explained that she got it for the Big Melanoma Clinic copies, out of lack of confidence in Dr. B's office. They had not demonstrated any professional courtesy, respect for patient intention, or concern for the other clinic's/patient's "need to know," or the fact that she was the most logical access to any of the above. They didn't care about anything but their rules.

Dr. B's office should have had a policy whereby positive pathology reports were given to another physician to evaluate, and arrange to call the patient. They should have offered a release at anytime when we were there together. They should have said that the Big Melanoma Clinic would need records and slides, and they would be glad to help expedite that. They could have offered Mom the slides, and asked that she follow up with the signed consent.

My mom is a wonderful sweet woman who has served in the medical community the majority of her life. The depiction above is more of a mother who was worried for her son than who she really is or how she normally acts. I am encouraged and proud of my mom because she has fully adopted a primarily raw, vegan lifestyle, and she is much healthier herself than she was at this time. To clarify, at the time, she was working in the medium-sized clinic in Seattle where this all started. My mom also accompanied us to nearly all of our appointments the first few months.

11/23/99   Mom, Nikki, and I had the first appointment with Dr. D, and we all liked him very much. He was quite upbeat and nice. The whole group at the Big Melanoma Clinic treated us with the utmost courtesy and concern. They were totally comfortable with the family visit.

11/23/99   *Doctor's notes: Initial visit schedule with Dr D, Big Melanoma Clinic Surgeon for wide excision and sentinel lymph node mapping of the mole excision area.*

12/2/99   I had the lymph mapping, another mole excised, and the wide excision on my back.

12/14/99   Mom, Nikki, and I went to my appointment to get results and have my stitches removed. The incisions looked fine and Dr. D took the stitches out. The pathology, however, was not good. One node (the sentinel) was positive, and Dr. D would have to do a full excision of the lymph nodes in the left axilla (armpit), which would leave me somewhat concave, permanently numb in some areas, and recuperating for weeks with limited mobility.

12/16/99 *Doctors notes: CT scan to clear the liver of cancer — negative.*

12/21/99 Consultation with oncologist, Dr. E, who suggested Interferon for one year with intravenous injections of 20 million units on Mondays and Fridays, followed by eleven months of 10 million units subcutaneously Mondays, Wednesdays, and Fridays. They also offered a randomized trial study treatment of a new vaccine, Melacine, plus lower doses of Interferon for a total of two years.

Mom, Nikki and I met with Dr. E, the oncologist. He told us that he and Dr. D had reviewed the pathology report, and felt that it should have been a 2.3 millimeter melanoma instead of a 1.14 millimeter, which is a substantial difference. The CT scan was fine. They recommended Interferon treatment, or the randomized study of Interferon, or Interferon and Melacine. He went over all the ramifications and adversities to the drugs, which were two year's worth of the worst fatigue and depression I could ever imagine, as well as possible destruction of other cells and hair loss, and such.

Dr. E informed us of the overall prognosis at this point. He indicated that he believed my chances were about 5% overall to live 10 or more years thus the title of this book. He also said that I likely had a 40% 5 year survival rate. If I choose to succom to the chemical treatments he was recommending, he felt I could improve my odds by 15% overall.

This was also the meeting when Dr. E informed us we would not be able to have children and that my racing career was over. Mom, Nikki, and I would always pray at these meetings, but this was one of the most difficult and, I believe, the only one we cried at.

After Dr. E left the room, we huddled together, wept, and prayed.

12/21/99   *Doctors notes: Second opinion of the original dermopathology suggested that it had been read incorrectly and was actually 2.3mm because it had actually followed a hair follicle down.* (see note at the end of the chronology addressing level and stage issues / contradiction)

12/27/99   I had surgery to have my whole auxiliary lymphatic system removed. I had a drain in for a week or so, and waited for the biopsy report until Thursday just before the New Year. Basically what that meant was they cut open my left armpit and cut all the lymph system out. At the time of this operation, I weighed 213 pounds.

> FIELD NOTES: This was just two days after we watched the *How to Eliminate Sickness* video (now called: God's Way to Ultimate Health). I remember lying on the bed waiting to be wheeled into the operation room, thinking to myself, "What on earth am I doing? I know this is wrong, but everyone around me wants me to do it. If I get out of this bed, my family will flip out and everyone will think I am crazy." In retrospect, and especially after going through the weeks that followed this surgery, I wish I would have gotten off that bed and walked out of the hospital!

This was really the start of the self-healing journey for us. I just wish I would have started just a little bit sooner. The encouragement and support from my family was important during this time, but the pressure to do what the doctors said was overwhelming. Our education did increase, as did our faith, in what we now know to be true.

| 1/4/00 | Appointments to have the drain taken out or checked, and results of the biopsy which were not available before the holiday. |

Doctor's notes: Post operative visit with Dr. D.

| 1/11/00 | I had an appointment with Dr. F, an oncologist. This appointment with Dr. F was both frustrating and enlightening. We explored the survival rates, actual causes of cancer (per standard medical assumptions) and carcinogen effects, the poor prognosis of recurrence, and the treatment options available. Even then, he would not give me more than a 60% chance of survival without high-dose Interferon, Melacine, or Interluken. These treatments would raise the survival chance to about 70-75%. He said they had no way to know if there were any more tumors until it could be too late. His advice included, primarily, the high-dose Interferon, and secondarily, the study with Interferon and Melacine. He did not know of another way to get the vaccine other than at the Big Melanoma Clinic. He did not think the consultant that group hired to do the research was of much value, stating that he or we could pull it right off the internet ourselves. He also believed in vitamin E, Selenium, and vitamin C combined with a healthy diet, but said they did not have data to prove that any diet helped. He said the Interluken, while given only a few months instead of a year or two, was so toxic it had a small chance of killing me while trying to kill the cancer. Dr. F actually got very hostile when I mentioned not taking the standard treatment, and Mom felt really bad because she had recommended Dr. F as a second source. |

| 1/13/00 | My initial visit with Dr. G, a naturopath. Dr. G recommended several dietary restrictions and several supplements. I started taking his list of supplements, which was about $600 per month. He also suggested a diet without red meat, dairy, or simple carbohydrates. He also suggested increasing seafood, soy, green tea, |

fruits, vegetables, legumes, whole grains, yams, squash, olive oil, nuts, and seeds. Dr. G recommended 20mg of melatonin at bedtime to slow growth of abnormal cells. I slowly quit taking all the supplements over a six-month period after starting. They just seemed like a waste of money, and only really applicable for someone who refused to change what they were eating. Since I was fully adopting a healthy diet and lifestyle, I didn't feel like I needed all those supplements.

> FIELD NOTES: I did eat seafood as a transitional food about once a quarter for the first year, but eventually lost the desire for it. That is better because there are some serious mercury issues with seafood. If you look on page 129 of *Eat to Live* by Dr. Joel Fuhrman, he identifies which types of seafood are known to be worse than others for the mercury issue. I am not advocating that you eat any seafood, but if you are going to use it as I did once in a while, then you should know as much as you can about it.

4/00   My first three-month visit. "All looks good." I had lost a lot of weight, and they said I was doing really well. "Whatever you are doing, keep it up."

7/00   "Wow," they said, "you have lost over forty pounds, you look great. Seriously, what are you doing? We don't need to see you for another six months."

1/9/01 One year follow-up visit with Dr. D. No evidence of recurrent melanoma. He agreed with our diet and lifestyle approach, but expressed concern that I may not be able to sustain the lifestyle long-term. This proved his wisdom, because we live in an unhealthy culture, but also proved that he didn't know me or the level of desire I have for life and my aspirations. "No need to come in every six months for these visits. See you in a year!" That final visit never did happen.

1/02   Final CAT scan which was, like the rest, clear. Lots of detail is missing in the chronology above. One stark omission is the dates and appointments with another dermatologist who I will refer to as Dr. H once I gather up the info. I saw him in three-month intervals for the first year, and then six months the second year. We did CAT scans every six months, but I need to dig up all the data on that as well.

I lost about forty pounds the first year, and then it seemed to level off for a year or more. Then I lost another twenty pounds, and I have pretty much stayed between 155-165 ever since.

CLARIFICATION:

The survival percentages quoted on 1/11/00 were from a different doctor in a different clinic, and this was the first visit where he had no prior knowledge of my situation. These survival estimates are radically different than the ones given to us by the Big Melanoma Clinic, and I do not know on what they are based. I assume it's a professional guess.

On 1/11/00, the doctor mentions "the fear of returning melanoma," which tends to be even more scary than a first diagnosis because it often returns internally, advances very fast, and attacks critical, high blood-flow organs such as the heart, brain, and lungs. This information was corroborated by the doctors at the Big Melanoma Clinic.

Throughout the first few years following my diagnosis, there was a lot of confusion on the actual level or stage of my diagnosis. We have documented proof that the various doctors did not agree in the staging, or established the level because of their process of reading the scans of the actual mole. These diagnoses are confused by different measurement types as well. The two types referred to in my story are Staging (stage 1 through 5, where 5 is the worst case), which is commonly used among many cancers, and Clark's Level (Clark's Level 1-5—see chart), which is specific to melanoma cancer. My diagnosis was a Stage 3 and Clark's Level 4, based on the information we have gathered. We were, however, told it was Stage 4 once it was confirmed that it had spread to the lymph system. There was also a discrepancy in the way the depth was measured because it was much deeper along a hair follicle than the rest of the mole. I also find the Clark's Level rather confusing because the cancer had spread, but the definitions for the levels don't specifically cover that type of situation.

FIELD NOTES: This whole thing makes me wonder what else I don't know? Or another way of putting it is, "What else am I totally clueless about?" This life change was so radical for us that we were profoundly impacted at the core of our belief system. We were not arrogant enough to think we knew it all, but this whole idea that the foods we were eating were actually causing the diseases was astounding. It made us wonder, and possibly opened ourselves up to the Spirit of Truth even more. Hopefully that has enabled us to more fully live the lives God intended for us because we are less likely to accept something "just because it has always been that way." I want to challenge you to question what you believe and verify that it is in full alignment with Truth. Thank God we have Truth as a frame of reference for everything in life.

Jerrod Sessler

After being given a five percent chance of surviving advanced-stage melanoma skin cancer, author and speaker Jerrod Sessler decided to take responsibility not only for his recovery but for his health as well. Jerrod's story is a riveting message of hope and healing that will inspire you. His delivery is full of energy and enthusiasm for the health message that has become his passion, a message that he says is very basic but much obscured by our culture. Jerrod speaks regularly on the topics of health, racing and faith.

Jerrod has earned multiple engineering degrees along with multiple certifications and recognitions from associations such as the *Small Business Administration*, *Entrepreneur Magazine*, the *International Franchise Association*, *Hallelujah Acres* and the *National Heritage Foundation*. Jerrod is an honored veteran and also serves as a PCO and volunteer lobbyist in his state and in Washington, DC.

Jerrod Sessler is a successful entrepreneur in business and serves in several non-profit foundations. He has also gained recognition as a successful NASCAR Driver.

Contact Jerrod:

Thank you for reading my book. I look forward to connecting with you and hearing your story. Contact me using one of the methods below.

Bonus Materials: www.FivePercentChance.com/bonus.htm

Facebook: http://www.facebook.com/pages/Jerrod-Sessler/94230561313

Twitter: "Sessler"

Web: www.hope4health.org; www.jerrodsessler.com; www.freggies.com; www.hometask.com

Support:

Contact Hallelujah Acres & ask for a Health Minister in your area. www.hacres.com or call 1-800-915-9355.